How to Prevent a Stroke

How to Prevent a Stroke

A COMPLETE RISK-REDUCTION PROGRAM

BY
Peggy Jo Donahue
and the Editors of ***PREVENTION*** ® Magazine

Mark L. Dyken, M.D., and Philip A. Wolf, M.D.,
Medical Advisers

Rodale Press, Emmaus, Pennsylvania

Excerpt from WINGS by Arthur Kopit. Copyright © 1978 by Arthur Kopit. Reprinted by permission of Hill and Wang, a division of Farrar, Straus and Giroux, Inc.

Printed in the United States of America

Book design by Denise Mirabello

Library of Congress Cataloging-in-Publication Data

Donahue, Peggy Jo.
    How to prevent a stroke.

    Includes index.
    1. Cerebrovascular diseases—Prevention—Popular works.
I. Prevention (Emmaus, Pa.) II. Title.
RC388.5.D63   1989   616.8'1   88-26355
ISBN 0–87857–781–5 hardcover
ISBN 0–87857–785–8 paperback

Distributed in the book trade by St. Martin's Press

2 4 6 8 10 9 7 5 3   hardcover
2 4 6 8 10 9 7 5 3   paperback

Notice

This book is intended as a reference volume only, not as a medical manual or a guide to self-treatment. If you suspect that you have a medical problem, we urge you to seek competent medical help. Keep in mind that nutritional and health needs vary from person to person, depending on age, sex, health status and total diet. The information here is intended to help you make informed decisions about your health, not as a substitute for any treatment that may have been prescribed by your doctor.

To my husband, Bill, my friend since childhood: Thanks for a lifetime of support, encouragement and love—from the mud puddle to the book.

and

To my mother and father, Herb and Peggy Ruetsch, for all their love.

Contents

Foreword

Injury or destruction of brain cells as a result of blockage or rupture of an artery to the brain usually occurs suddenly and often without warning. In the past, the stroke seemed to come "out of the blue," so it was viewed as an "accident," an unexpected and unpredictable event. It's no coincidence that an old-fashioned medical term for stroke is cerebrovascular accident.

It is now known, however, that stroke is no accident of nature but the *predictable* outcome of a chain of events set in motion many years before, and that this chain can be interrupted and risk of stroke substantially reduced. Stroke is often an affliction of later life and is particularly dreaded by the elderly, who often fear the disability and loss of independence from brain injury more than death itself. As more people are living into the eighth and ninth decades of life, when risk of stroke is greatest, the challenge to prevent this dread disease increases.

Fortunately, there is cause for optimism and hope. Factors that predispose to stroke have been identified, and modification of these risk factors can be accomplished. Over the past 20 years, numerous scientific studies, particularly trials of lowering blood pressure in hypertensives, have cut stroke rates in half. Death rates from stroke have been falling by 5 percent per year throughout the world; since 1968, deaths from stroke in the United States have fallen by 50 percent.

But much remains to be done, and fortunately, the tools are available. In *How to Prevent a Stroke*, Peggy Jo Donahue outlines the current state of knowledge of stroke prevention and does so in a manner that is readable and easily understood. The book also contains important information for stroke survivors and their families. In particular, the appendix should provide much-needed assistance in locating agencies and persons who provide services to improve the quality of life after stroke.

Further scientific research is needed to identify other risk factors and to develop preventive strategies for stroke. Measures to reduce the damage to the brain at the time of the acute stroke are also under active investigation.

It is clear, however, that prevention, not improved treatment of stroke patients, holds the key to conquest of stroke.

Mark L. Dyken, M.D.   Philip A. Wolf, M.D.

Acknowledgments

My thanks go first to my mother, Margaret Deegan Ruetsch, who taught me how to write. It was her stroke-warning attack that led to my interest in writing this book.

Equally heartfelt thanks go to Mark L. Dyken, M.D., and Philip A. Wolf, M.D., my two medical advisers on the book. They spent hours of their valuable time educating me, pointing me in the right directions and carefully reading every page of the manuscript.

Thanks also to my "doctor friends" Christine Stabler, M.D., Christopher Roberts, M.D., and Charles Norelli, M.D., who shared with me their day-to-day experiences caring for people at risk for or recovering from stroke. And thanks to Pat Kasell, coordinator of the Courage Stroke Network at the Courage Center in Minneapolis, who also spent hours helping me learn about the many services available to stroke survivors.

My great thanks go out to the stroke survivors and caregivers associated with the Courage Stroke Network. It is their insights that give the stroke survival chapters their warmth and accuracy.

And finally, to the people at Rodale Press who helped bring this book into existence: Bill Gottlieb, for his sympathetic and supportive ear; Ellen Michaud, my editor, for her careful shepherding of the book through the Rodale system; and Roberta Mulliner and her staff for the million and one tasks involved in getting this manuscript physically ready for printing. A special thanks to Rodale head librarian Janet Glassman and library staffers Lynn Donches, Tawna Clelan, Liz Wolbach, Doreen Keyser and others who helped in so many ways to be sure I had the latest in medical information about stroke.

Introduction

The Lessons of a Sunday Morning

When my mother was 48 years old, she suffered what we were all told was a "mini-stroke."

She was making breakfast for the family on a Sunday morning when she started to lose feeling in her right hand and was unable to grip the handle of a frying pan. She sat down uneasily at the kitchen table and tried to flex her fingers.

My father, who was also in the kitchen at the time, remembers that she began to slur her words and that the right side of her face started to droop. My mother didn't know this was happening—not until my dad pointed it out. Then they went to the hospital emergency room where my mother was told she'd had a stroke warning episode called a transient ischemic attack (TIA)—what some people call a "mini-stroke." Although not a genuine stroke, the doctor explained, a TIA was her body's warning that she was highly vulnerable to the real thing.

One woman's story.

A TIA was her body's warning.

My mother's doctor also explained to her what the risk factors are for having a stroke. Smoking cigarettes was among them. So she decided then and there to give up the habit. It was a difficult task for this almost three-pack-a-day smoker who had grown up with romantic images of movie stars offering one another a cigarette. But she never looked back. And she never smoked again.

"What scared me the most," says this articulate and talented teacher, "was the prospect of losing my ability to speak and communicate."

But my mother was one of the lucky ones. She got a warning. It convinced her to give up smoking and get the kind of medical treatment and follow-up monitoring that can be crucial to stroke prevention. She never did have a full-fledged stroke. The weakness on her right side and her speech problems eventually cleared up, and she's healthy and free of stroke symptoms to this day—12 years later.

My mother had to have a frightening strokelike attack before she would do something to change her stroke-bound course, but you don't.

It doesn't have to happen to you.

You don't because this book will tell you why so many of us—the majority of us, in fact—are on that same crash course as my mother. And it will tell you how to get off.

How to Prevent a Stroke

Stroke prevention involves three simple steps:

1. Gaining knowledge. You need to know what a stroke is, what's going on in your body to let it occur, and what the consequences are. You also need to know what's putting you at risk for having a stroke. Some risk factors, like your age, sex and family history, can't be changed,

of course. But others, like smoking, poor eating habits, lack of exercise or undetected high blood pressure, can.

It's also crucial that you understand the body's most compelling warning signal—the transient ischemic attack (TIA), like the one my mother had. Many people ignore these truly frightening physical signals, chalking them up to fatigue or growing older. That is a dangerous course to follow.

Three simple steps to a stroke-free life.

2. Taking action. This is a key to preventing a stroke from happening to you. Things that you can do yourself are eliminating some bad habits like smoking or drinking, changing your diet, increasing your physical activity and keeping your blood pressure under control. That's the heart of what this book is all about. Before you ever need to face an emergency room, complicated, expensive tests and myriad medications—you and your own body can be working to change the conditions that make you a sitting duck for a stroke. We'll give you the tools to get started.

3. Learning how the medical world works. The sophisticated world of stroke research has produced many complex preventive treatments which doctors use every day. You need to know what those treatments are so that you can discuss them knowledgeably with your health care providers and decide whether or not they're for you.

Knowledge is your most important weapon.

Most of these treatments involve drugs and/or surgery. That's why *How to Prevent a Stroke* provides you with a complete resource guide to the drugs currently being used to prevent strokes. We'll also discuss the pros and cons of several preventive but controversial surgical techniques that are sometimes performed on people at high risk for having a stroke.

What stroke prevention is all about is your getting in the driver's seat and taking control of a body that doesn't have to be slowed down by an inevitable disease process. It's you, learning how to improve the quality of your life through positive change. It's you, learning to deal with a medical world grown increasingly complex.

You're in charge.

It's you, in charge. You, in control.

Part 1

Are You at Risk?

Chapter 1

Stroke: When the Brain Is Starved of Blood

Suddenly, the things you take for granted, like tying your shoes, buttoning your coat and getting out of bed, are beyond your control.

You must be helped to walk, eat and go to the bathroom. You have trouble comprehending what people are saying—it sounds like another language. Worse still, you can't seem to speak in words that people understand. Sometimes you cry uncontrollably, even when you don't feel like crying. You can see your family and friends struggling to maintain a normal relationship with you.

It's easy to understand why some people say they'd rather die than wake up one day and cope with the life-shattering disabilities that can accompany a stroke.

The National Stroke Association (NSA) estimates that between 500,000 and 600,000 people a year in the United States suffer a stroke. Of those,

Do you prefer death? Or disability?

more than 150,000 die, estimates the American Heart Association (AHA). And, although it doesn't receive nearly as much attention or press coverage, stroke is the third leading cause of death in the United States, outranked only by heart disease and cancer.

Stroke is also the leading cause of adult disability in America. In fact, says the NSA, there are two to three million people living in this country with stroke aftereffects.

Of people who survive a stroke, nearly two-thirds may actually be handicapped, estimates the National Institute of Neurological and Communicative Disorders and Stroke (NINCDS), the leading federal agency responsible for stroke research.

Two-thirds of all stroke survivors may be disabled.

Their handicaps include the inability to control bodily functions, the inability to walk, impaired vision, impaired speech and/or comprehension, depression, memory loss—even paralysis on one side of the body.

Of every 100 people who survive the acute illness phase of stroke, reports the U.S. Food and Drug Administration, only about 10 will ever return to work without impairment.

And as if that's not hard enough for the stroke survivor to bear, think about the effect that these handicaps can have on the survivors' family relationships, friendships, sense of independence and mobility. Think about the strain that constant care of a stroke survivor places on his or her caregivers. And think about the financial worries produced by the uninsured expenses that inevitably crop up.

The effect on your family is difficult to bear.

Grim, isn't it? Maybe that's why stroke is one subject some people would rather not talk about. And it could also be one of the reasons stroke doesn't receive the attention that heart disease does. After a heart attack, most people can still walk, talk, think and control their bodily functions. And about 80 percent of those wo survive a heart attack can return to work within three months, according to the AHA.

That's all the bad news. Now we'll tell you the good news: Death rates from stroke have been declining at a rate of about 6 percent a year since 1973, according to the AHA. During the 1940s and 1950s, in comparison, the rate was declining by only about 1 percent a year. So we've increased our chances of surviving a stroke more than six-fold in less than 50 years. And the difference is stroke *prevention.*

Prevention has increased your chance of surviving a stroke sixfold.

Americans are doing a lot more to detect, control and prevent high blood pressure, one of the major causes of so many strokes. We're also doing more to prevent heart disease, another factor that puts you at high risk of having a stroke. How? Through better diet and less sedentary living, and by giving up smoking, among other things. In addition, doctors are also helping to prevent stroke deaths through better diagnostic tests and treatments.

Better diagnostic tests help prevent stroke.

Yet we still have a long way to go. Stroke touches one in ten families. The stroke death rate is still unacceptably high, as are the disability figures. Making sure that you're not one of those statistics is what this book is all about.

What Happens in Your Body to Let a Stroke Occur?

A stroke is a sudden disruption in the flow of blood that supplies life-sustaining oxygen and nutrients to your brain. Deprived of blood for even a short time, the affected brain cells either become damaged or die. Body functions—moving your limbs, for example, or speaking—that were controlled by those damaged or dead brain cells are now impaired. Sometimes permanently.

But even though we talk about the "suddenness" of a stroke and the "swiftness" with which it can cause damage, a stroke is usually due to a disease that has been slowly building up in your body most of your life.

Clogged arteries set the stage.

It's the disease called *atherosclerosis*, which is a form of *arteriosclerosis*—sometimes called hardening of the arteries. You may be familiar with it as the culprit behind many forms of heart disease. Well, it's also the bad guy behind most strokes.

When atherosclerosis occurs, for example, it means that deposits of fat, cholesterol and other substances have built up on the inner walls of your arteries, causing them to narrow and inhibit the free flow of blood.

As these deposits build, your arteries also become hard and constricted instead of supple. That makes them more vulnerable to a blood clot forming and getting stuck there, blocking off the blood supply completely. If that happens in one of the arteries that supplies blood to your heart, you'll have a heart attack. If it happens in one the arteries supplying blood to your brain, you'll have a stroke.

What are the chances that you have atherosclerosis? The AHA says more than one of every four Americans has heart or blood vessel disease (which includes strokes)—over 63 million people. And the single biggest cause of these diseases is atherosclerosis.

The diet that's killing Americans.

But why do so many of us have this life-threatening disease building up in our bodies? It's a complex disease that has many causes, say the scientists studying it. One of the main causes, researchers have come to discover, is a diet high in cholesterol and saturated fats—the kind of diet most Americans live on. Such a diet causes you to build up too much cholesterol in your bloodstream, and this fatty substance contributes to atherosclerosis.

Of course, there are also many other factors that combine with atherosclerosis to raise your risk of having a stroke, most prominently high blood pressure. We'll discuss them more fully in the next chapter.

The Three Major Ways a Stroke Occurs

A stroke occurs when an artery supplying crucial oxygen and nutrients via the blood to your brain clogs or bursts.

Without blood-supplied oxygen and glucose (the energy or fuel your brain uses to operate), brain cells simply shut down and refuse to work. Except in rare and special circumstances, in approximately 3 to 10 minutes they die. Here's how brain shutdown most frequently occurs.

The thrombotic stroke. This is one of the most common forms of stroke. It occurs when an artery supplying blood to the brain is blocked by a blood clot called a *thrombus*, which forms inside the artery.

Blood clots form most frequently in arteries that are—you guessed it—damaged because of atherosclerosis. Why? Because blood is "programmed" to flow through the arteries and veins, but to clot when it comes in contact with foreign matter. Those atherosclerotic fatty deposits are definitely considered foreign matter by your blood.

The embolic stroke. Another common cause of strokes is when a blood clot called an *embolus* is carried in the bloodstream and becomes wedged in one of the arteries supplying blood to the brain. Often this clot comes from a diseased heart.

The hemorrhagic stroke. The third major way a stroke occurs is when an artery in or on the surface of the brain bursts and floods the surrounding tissue with blood—a *hemorrhage*. The brain cells nourished by this artery can no longer do their job. And the blood flooding into or near the brain can interfere with the way the brain functions. This is the most severe form of stroke, and it's more likely to occur when a person suffers from a combination of atherosclerosis and high blood pressure.

Your brain cells go on strike.

High blood pressure and atherosclerosis are an explosive combination.

The brain can heal itself.

The amount of damage inflicted by any of these kinds of stroke depends on a number of factors. One of the most remarkable things that happens when someone has a stroke is that often the body attempts a repair job by causing small neighboring arteries to get larger and take over the work of the damaged artery. In this way, some brain cells that are not yet dead may recover. That's why some people who have paralyzed muscles, speech loss, impaired memories and other stroke effects may eventually see improvement. A muscle may regain strength, speech may return.

Now you know why and how most strokes occur. In the next section, we'll explain how your body reacts to this calamitous event.

The Stroke Emergency: Your Body Reacts

An experience in chaos.

In Arthur Kopit's play *Wings*, we are taken into the strange world of a woman named Emily Stilson, who has suffered a stroke. "The moment of a stroke, even a relatively minor one, and its immediate aftermath, are an experience in chaos," writes Kopit, whose father suffered a severe stroke just before Kopit began to research his play.

Nothing "makes sense" after a stroke.

"Nothing at all makes sense. Nothing except perhaps this overwhelming disorientation will be remembered by the victim. The stroke usually happens suddenly. It is a catastrophe."

" . . . *trees clouds houses*
mostly planes flashing past,
images without words, utter
disarray disbelief, never seen
this kind of thing before!

"Where am I? How'd I get
here?
My leg (What's my leg?)
feels wet arms . . . wet too,
belly same chin nose
everything (Where are they

taking me?) something sticky
(What has happened to my
plane?) feel something
sticky

"Doors! Too many doors!
"Must have . . . fallen cannot
. . . move at all sky . . .
(Gliding!) dark cannot . . .
talk (Feels as if I'm gliding!)."

A mind that falls from
the sky.

(Emily Stilson, stroke survivor in *Wings*)

Kopit learned a great deal about the kinds of
brain disorders many stroke survivors experience
through discussions with a stroke therapist. The
therapist, who had herself recovered from a head
injury sustained in a traffic accident, shared with
Kopit vivid descriptions of what it was like to live
in the world of the brain-damaged.

A gifted therapist shares
her life with a playwright.

This therapist worked at the rehabilitation
hospital where Kopit's father was sent. Kopit spent
a lot of time there talking to her and observing two
female stroke survivors who became the composite character of Emily Stilson.

Kopit's play serves to illustrate the often-hor-
rible confusion that accompanies so many stroke
attacks. This mental confusion, though, is but one
of the many ways your body could possibly react
to a stroke. Here's a description of what else can
occur.

When Catastrophe Strikes: Paralysis

When most people think of the effects of stroke,
they think of being paralyzed on one side of the
body. It's often the most visible sign that a stroke
has occurred. But why?

Usually a stroke occurs only in one side, or
hemisphere, of the brain. Since the left and right
sides of our brains control different bodily functions, only certain portions of bodily function are

lost. The most obvious manifestation of this is one-sided paralysis. The left hemisphere of the brain controls function on the right side of the body and the right hemisphere controls function on the left side of the body.

Your body can become a prison.

Whether paralysis has occurred on the right or left side, it creates tremendous problems. Here's how gifted choreographer Agnes de Mille, who suffered paralysis on the right side of her body after a massive stroke, describes the experience: "Half of me was imprisoned in the other half. The dead side seemed unaccountably heavy, gigantically heavy and restrained with bonds. Cement. Wood. When I rolled in bed and tried to get onto my right, or dead, side, I rolled against a dyke of unfeeling matter which I lacked the strength to go over or rise against."

Physical therapists and nurses go to work as quickly as they can to try to alleviate the consequences of unfeeling limbs, says Conn Foley, M.D., coauthor of *The Stroke Fact Book* and medical director at the Jewish Institute for Geriatric Care, Long Island, New York. Those consequences include bedsores from lying on the paralyzed side, blood clots, pneumonia and other complications that can result from prolonged bed rest.

Gentle movements prevent damage.

In addition to having an arm or a leg with no feeling in it, the stroke survivor loses pain sensation. Moreover, a totally flaccid arm can cause the shoulder joint to become deformed because the "dead weight" of an arm can pull the bone out of its normal position in the socket. A leg allowed to turn outward can alter the hip joint, making it impossible for the person to relearn to walk. By passively moving and gently exercising the limbs, therapists try to prevent these things.

Is it a hand? Or the hind leg of a donkey?

Another consequence of paralysis is that some people develop a nerve disorder which involves jerky uncontrolled movement. Agnes de Mille remembers: "There were . . . irrational and insane jerkings which I was not aware of. My hand would fly out and encounter, well, whatever there was to encounter ... training that right hand to do the most primitive bidding was like training a wild animal ... it was not my hand. It was not anybody's hand. It could have been the hind leg of a donkey."

But paralysis is only the most obvious sign of the kind of stroke sustained. Here are some of the other kinds of injuries that occur in left- and right-brain strokes.

Left-Brain Strokes: Speech and Language

In addition to paralysis on the right side of the body, a person with a left-brain stroke injury is likely to have problems with speech and language. This is called aphasia.

A person with aphasia can lose the ability to speak lucidly—his words come out like gibberish. Or an aphasic hears people speaking to him, but the words sound like nonsense.

Although an aphasic stroke survivor loses the ability to make sense of language, the injury usually does not affect intelligence. Aphasics remain mentally alert, even though their speech may be jumbled or incoherent and they may not be able to comprehend words spoken to them. "It's like being in a foreign land, unable to speak or understand the native tongue," reports NINCDS.

Jumbled speech does not mean a jumbled mind.

To the horror of many stroke survivors, however, those around them may not realize that intelligence has remained intact. Because survivors cannot make sense when they speak or write, or cannot comprehend or correctly answer questions, many people patronize aphasics and treat them as if they were mentally incompetent—or shout at them as if they were hard of hearing.

What comes out of your mouth is not the same word that left your brain.

Emily Stilson, the stroke survivor in the play *Wings*, is aphasic. Doctors ask her to name the first president of the United States, and she thinks that she has replied "Washington." But the doctors keep repeating the question until it becomes clear that what's coming out of her mouth is not "Washington." The second doctor says to the first: "I don't think she hears herself."

At other times, Stilson hears people at the hospital speaking to her. This is a sample of what she hears: "Are we moving you too fast? Mustlian pottid or blastiigrate, no not that way this, that's fletchit gottit careful now."

Ears that don't work.

There are two categories of aphasia that we've described here. The first is *expressive aphasia*, where patients know what they want to say but cannot find the words they need. They have thoughts but can't recall or organize the language to express them. The other is *receptive aphasia*, where patients hear the voice or see the print but cannot make sense of the words. Even though they may talk a great deal, they often don't make sense. Victims of receptive aphasia often substitute sounds in their words, making them unintelligible to others.

Your ability to make decisions may be impaired.

People who suffer from left-brain strokes also tend to be slow, cautious and disorganized when approaching an unfamiliar problem. A once-decisive, highly organized executive, for example, suddenly looks to his wife for approval of things as simple as putting on his shirt. Even after she gives him support and positive feedback, he still feels anxious and hesitant about his ability to perform simple tasks.

Right-Brain Strokes: Spatial-Perceptual Tasks

In addition to paralysis on the left side of the body, the right-brain stroke survivor is more likely to show difficulty with spatial-perceptual tasks. This means he will have trouble judging distance, size, position and rate of movement, as well as the relation of parts to wholes. We all do this sometimes. Have you ever seen a person driving a car hesitate to pass through a narrow space because he thinks his car may get stuck? *You* can see he has plenty of room, but *he* cannot.

For the stroke survivor, these spatial-perceptual errors are likely to happen more frequently and consistently. He may not be able to steer a wheelchair through a large doorway without bumping the frame. He may confuse the inside and outside of his clothes, or have difficulty knowing when he's standing upright and when he's leaning. Someone with even minor spatial-perceptual difficulties will not be safe driving a car.

You may not be able to judge distances.

The person with a right-brain stroke will also tend to be impulsive and proceed too fast, behaving as if he were unaware of his inability to do certain things, like perform spatial-perceptual tasks. For this reason, he may attempt to do things that are not within his abilities and may be unsafe. He may try to walk across the room without support, and fall. Or he may attempt to drive, and injure himself and others. This kind of stroke survivor is usually a poor judge of his own abilities.

You may become impulsive.

Other General Effects of Strokes

Many stroke effects hit all kinds of stroke survivors, regardless of which side of their brains were affected. People who have suffered both right- and left-brain strokes can develop one-sided neglect, although the right-brain stroke survivor suffers more from this. One-sided neglect means that the stroke survivor becomes unaware of things on the damaged side of his body. He may not even recognize his own arm and leg as parts of his body. In addition, he may not look to the left (or right) of a page and could miss information printed there.

Among other general effects of strokes are problems with social judgment. A sharp dresser may become sloppy about his appearance. A shy person may become aggressive or a quiet person boisterous. An interesting storyteller may become boring and repetitive. These traits may strain

Your personality may change.

stroke survivors' relationships with those closest to them, who now find them annoying.

A stroke survivor may also have an array of complicated memory problems. "I would tell my wife to call our daughter, ask her if she could bring us our mail and stay to dinner. All she'd remember was to call my daughter," the spouse of a typical stroke patient might complain. Another patient might have trouble remembering new information, even though her recall of information from the past is fine. "I can tell you what I was doing the day Pearl Harbor was bombed, but don't ask me what I had for breakfast," a stroke survivor might tell you.

You may even forget what you had for breakfast.

Another might lose the ability to apply what has been learned in one setting to another. He may have learned in the hospital how to transfer himself from wheelchair to bed but won't be able to do it at home, in a different bed and room. Or some stroke survivors may simply not be able to remember phone numbers, appointments or names of new friends.

A stroke survivor may also switch from crying to laughing for no apparent reason. Often the crying or laughing doesn't indicate sadness or happiness—the person may just have lost the ability to control his emotions because of physical damage to the brain. Coping with these emotional outbursts can be embarrassing and difficult for the stroke survivor's family, because it's sometimes hard to tell if the person is expressing genuine feelings and emotions. Since many stroke survivors are truly depressed about their condition, for example, they may sometimes cry for very valid reasons.

You may chuckle at a funeral. Or sob at a party.

This explicit description of some of the many complex effects that a stroke can have on human performance is not meant to scare but to inform and motivate, because there *is* a way to keep these things from happening. So let's move on and see what puts you at risk for a stroke to begin with.

Chapter 2

What Puts You at Risk for Stroke?

Phil lay in a deep sleep, not yet medically stable from the massive stroke he had suffered the day before. The monitors beeped, tracing his heartbeat in emerald green lines across the screen. Oxygen hissed from a transparent tube in his nose. Outside his hospital room, his wife and children talked with the doctor. Although deeply worried about Phil, they were also visibly angry. Because Phil had been warned that this could happen.

An angry family.

He had been warned that tests showed he was suffering from high blood pressure and heart disease, two major risk factors for stroke. Yet he had refused to take medication to lower his blood pressure. And, even though cigarette smoking and unhealthy diet clearly aggravated his heart problems, he had refused all encouragement from his family to lose weight and quit smoking. His son had offered to start a walking program with him. His daughter had found him a smoking cessation class that worked for a lot of people.

But Phil hadn't listened. To anyone.

Jean, however, did. When her doctor warned her that clogged arteries, high blood pressure, smoking and excess weight made her a perfect target for a heart attack or a stroke, she and her husband *both* signed up for a local smoking cessation class and attacked the necessary diet and exercise changes on their own.

A woman who turned her life around.

Soon they were walking and bicycling and had a shelf full of new recipe books instructing them how to prepare low-fat, low-calorie meals. By her doctor's next visit, Jean had lost 20 pounds and was completely off cigarettes. Stroke was probably no longer a part of her future.

Let's face it. There's a little bit of Phil and Jean in all of us, isn't there? There's the stubborn Phil part—denying that a problem may exist or that it will affect us, incapable of change, undaunted by the grim litany of diseases our doctors rattle off to us. But there's also the sensible Jean part—eager to learn how to prevent health problems, earnest in our desire to change, optimistic that it's worth trying.

Strokes are easier to prevent than to treat.

And when it comes to preventing strokes, you owe it to yourself to let the Jean side of your personality win out. Why? Because even those in the forefront of stroke research admit that it's still much easier to prevent a stroke than to treat a brain that's been damaged by one.

"There are really two important issues here," says Philip A. Wolf, M.D., professor of neurology at Boston University School of Medicine. "The first issue has to do with the brain's extreme vulnerability to lack of oxygen, which is cut off when a stroke occurs. Irreversible damage happens after only 4 to 5 minutes. The parts of the brain that die cannot regenerate," says Dr. Wolf, who is also the principal stroke scientist for the Framingham Heart Study, a highly respected examination of over 5,000 people that has told Americans what factors put them at risk for cardiovascular diseases like heart attack and stroke.

"The second issue is that, although we've made some headway in limiting the damage a stroke causes or in facilitating recovery, it hasn't been much. A stroke can still rob a person of his human characteristics of speech, memory and movement. One becomes a shadow of oneself," observes Dr. Wolf.

A stroke can rob you of your humanity.

All of which leads Mark L. Dyken, M.D., past chairman of the American Heart Association's Stroke Council and chairman of the Department of Neurology at Indiana University, to say "We're all convinced that the best way to fight strokes is to prevent them from happening in the first place."

That's why experts like Dr. Wolf have spent years poring over statistics compiled from large, representative populations of Americans to see which of them develop strokes. They look at the people who fall prey to stroke and they look at those who stay healthy. What distinguishes each group? Who and how many among them had high blood pressure? Heart disease? Diabetes? Who was overweight, smoked cigarettes or drank excessively? What they find out tells Americans which health problems, diseases and lifestyle habits put us most at risk for having a stroke.

But does knowing what puts Americans at risk—and working to reduce those risk factors—really have an effect on how many people suffer a stroke?

The answer is yes! The American Heart Association (AHA) issued a stroke risk factors statement in 1971, for example, that detailed what researchers had learned could put Americans at risk for stroke. Soon after, the death rate due to stroke started to decline. Today, researchers can proudly say that death from stroke has been cut in half.

Stroke deaths began to decline.

But some experts have questioned whether the lower stroke death rate might have more to do with the fact that doctors are better at keeping people alive after they've had a stroke. Does it?

The people of Rochester, Minnesota, say no. They have been studied extensively for many years by researchers at the Mayo Clinic, located there, and have provided doctors with some of the best information to date on who and how many people are afflicted by strokes.

An entire town cut its stroke rate in half.

In a study performed there, for example, researchers found that the incidence of new cases of stroke has declined in every five-year period since 1950. The total decline has been over 50 percent since 1950—a statistic supported by a shorter national survey of stroke incidence performed by researchers at the National Institute of Neurological and Communicative Disorders and Stroke (NINCDS).

Knowledge can help you prevent stroke.

All these statistics and figures lead to one pretty sure conclusion: Learning the risk factors and doing something about them can prevent a stroke. So let's begin by looking at the most important—and mostly preventable—risk factors for stroke.

High Blood Pressure: Public Enemy #1

Ask any doctor what's the single most important thing you can do to prevent a stroke and you'll get one sure answer: Keep your blood pressure levels below 140/90. (See the section, "What Do the Numbers Mean?" on page 36.) As risk factors go, high blood pressure, or hypertension, has two potent strikes against it: It has a dangerously powerful link to strokes and it affects millions of Americans—almost one in three American adults.

Lower blood pressure may be the key.

Dr. Wolf and the researchers at Framingham have found that the risk of having a stroke is directly related to how high your blood pressure is. The higher blood pressure gets, the more risk. Women are just as vulnerable as men, and the elderly don't escape either. Up through the eighth and ninth decades of life, it's just as important to control hypertension as it is at younger ages.

What is it that makes high blood pressure such a lethal risk factor for strokes? Let's look first at what blood pressure is. Your heart pumps blood through your arteries and veins to supply oxygen and nutrients throughout your body. The force of the blood against those blood vessels creates pressure. Increased blood pressure injures the lining of the arteries and hastens the development of atherosclerosis or stroke.

When a doctor listens to your blood pressure, he records two numbers—120/80, for example. The higher number is your systolic pressure, and it represents the amount of pressure in your arteries when your heart beats. The lower number is diastolic pressure. It represents the amount of pressure in your arteries when your heart relaxes between heartbeats. So, a reading of 120/80 would mean your systolic pressure is 120 and your diastolic pressure is 80.

When the pressure of blood in your arteries becomes elevated and stays that way, you've developed hypertension—high blood pressure. No one knows what causes most cases of high blood pressure, although drugs such as oral contraceptives, decongestant nose drops, anti-inflammatories, estrogens, steroids and medications that contain sodium have been known to trigger the problem.

Drugs—even nose drops—can cause the problem.

But doctors do know a lot about the *effects* of that increased pressure. Your heart, for one thing, has to work harder to push blood through the arteries to meet your body's needs. Like any other muscle that's put through a tough workout, your heart starts to get larger. But a heart isn't like a bicep. When your heart becomes greatly enlarged, it stops working as well as it should. And a badly functioning heart increases your risk of stroke.

High blood pressure is also hard on your arteries. The strain of elevated pressure causes them to become scarred, inelastic and hard. So instead of being as flexible as cooked pasta, they're more like a rubber hose. That's why hypertension aggravates

Too much pressure can turn an artery into a rubber hose.

atherosclerosis, the disease that narrows your arteries and is behind so many strokes. Clearly, arteries that are damaged by hypertension and narrowed by atherosclerosis have a much harder time expanding and contracting to promote a smooth and steady flow of blood—with its vital nutrients and oxygen—to your brain. If a clot forms or gets lodged in a damaged artery, you could have a stroke. Or a damaged artery in your brain could burst, causing the kind of stroke called a cerebral hemorrhage.

There are no symptoms to warn you.

But if you can intervene and get your blood pressure down to normal before it severely damages your arteries, then you're way ahead of the game. The longer you have undetected hypertension, the worse off you are, doctors say. That's why it's so important to have your blood pressure

Should You Use a Home Blood Pressure Machine?

What's the advantage of measuring your blood pressure at home? If you currently have normal blood pressure but have a family history of elevated levels that makes you more likely to inherit the condition, a machine could help you detect it sooner than if you wait to go to your doctor.

And if you already have high blood pressure, taking periodic readings reassures you that your efforts to control it through diet, exercise or drugs are working. The American Heart Association (AHA) says that such reassurance encourages many people to stay on their treatment program.

Moreover, studies have shown that home readings can give a more accurate picture of an individual's blood pressure than the reading obtained in the doctor's office, since it is possible that anxiety at the doctor's office could cause your blood pressure to rise temporarily.

If you decide to buy a home blood pressure

checked regularly. High blood pressure doesn't hurt, so you can't wait for "signs" of it to appear before doing something. For this reason, it's often called the silent killer.

But does detecting and aggressively treating hypertension really cause fewer strokes? Yes. In fact, many doctors think that the main reason the stroke death rate has declined so rapidly in recent years is because hypertension is being detected and controlled so much more effectively. Drugs, life-style changes—losing weight, curbing salt in-take—and public education programs that have made us more aware of the importance of blood pressure checkups have all played a role, scientists believe.

In 1982, a program called the Hypertension Detection and Follow-up Program reported what

Controlling high blood pressure means controlling stroke.

machine, look for one that's easy to use, advises the AHA. A machine with a digital readout is a good choice, since you don't need to fiddle with the stethoscope or learn to listen for the specific sounds of your blood pressure, says Edward R. Pinckney, M.D., author of *Do-It-Yourself Medical Testing.* The machine does that for you.

Accuracy is also an important factor. Digital electronic models need to be adjusted at least once a year by a trained technician, who is usually available through the medical supply house where you purchase your equipment.

When you first get a home blood pressure machine, make sure you ask the salesperson how to use it, or ask your doctor to give you a hand. And be sure to get a machine that includes written instructions on how to use it and care for it properly.

For more information on home blood pressure machines, send for the pamphlet called *Buying and Caring for Home Blood Pressure Equipment* from the American Heart Association, Box RP, 7320 Greenville Avenue, Dallas, TX 75231.

happened to the stroke incidence rate when people with hypertension were aggressively treated. The program divided almost 11,000 mildly and moderately hypertensive people into two groups. One group was given what the program called *stepped care*, an intensive approach to treating hypertension in which people were carefully treated and monitored to ensure that they achieved the best possible control over their disease. The second group was simply referred to medical care sources in the community, without any follow-up.

After five years, the difference between the number of strokes suffered in each group was marked. The stepped-care group suffered many fewer than those in the other group. And that included men and women of all ages and even those who had evidence of long-standing hypertension. In fact, the risk of dying from stroke and other cardiovascular diseases in the stepped-care group was almost the same as that of the general U.S. population. It's almost as if stepped care eliminated the risk of hypertension.

Aggressive monitoring and treatment practically eliminate the risk.

Heart Disease: Public Enemy #2

If hypertension is your number one enemy in the fight to root out stroke, then heart disease is its grim accomplice. People with heart disease, even if they don't have high blood pressure, have twice the overall risk of stroke as people with healthy hearts. There are several forms of heart disease that seem to increase stroke risk the most. Here's a list.

Heart disease doubles your risk of stroke.

Coronary heart disease. This is the form of heart disease that triples your risk of having a stroke. Coronary heart disease—one form of which is angina—means that the arteries going to your heart are clogged and narrowed by atherosclerosis. Blood has a hard time flowing through, and if a coronary artery becomes severely obstructed or the blood supply is cut off, part of the heart muscle dies, causing a heart attack.

Why do people with coronary heart disease suffer more strokes than people without it? Because if your heart's arteries are clogged, doctors suspect, there's a good chance that the arteries supplying your brain are getting clogged, too.

Congestive heart failure. This means that your heart is so damaged and weakened it can't handle its job, which is to circulate blood through your body. When that happens, circulation slows and blood returning to your heart backs up, causing congestion, which can make your legs and ankles swell. Sometimes your lungs collect fluid, too, making it difficult to breathe.

A heart that doesn't work.

What causes your heart to become damaged and weak? Some people's hearts are damaged by rheumatic fever. Others sustain damage during a heart attack. Still others are hurt by atherosclerosis or high blood pressure. There's an even greater risk of stroke with congestive heart failure than with coronary heart disease.

Left ventricular hypertrophy. *Hypertrophy* means "excessively enlarged or thickened." And this overdevelopment of the muscle on the left side of the heart, which doctors can detect through an electrocardiogram, is usually a sign of prolonged or severe hypertension. People with this problem have more than five or six times the risk of stroke as those without it.

An enlarged heart means you increase your risk of stroke at least fivefold.

Irregular heartbeats, especially atrial fibrillation. Irregular rhythms of the heart, especially a condition called atrial fibrillation, greatly increase your risk for stroke. Atrial fibrillation, in which your heart quivers instead of beats, increases your risk of stroke to more than six times that of a person without it. Why? When your heart quivers, the blood isn't completely pumped out of its upper chambers, and the blood that remains tends to clot. If one of those clots breaks loose, travels to your brain and blocks an artery, it causes the kind of stroke called a cerebral embolism.

This is why the AHA recommends that all

Americans be regularly checked for these kinds of heart problems.

Extra Red Blood Cells: Public Enemy #3

Even a moderate increase in the number of red blood cells your blood contains can put you at a greater risk of stroke. This has been confirmed in several studies. Why? Extra red blood cells increase the thickness of the blood, making it more likely that clots will occur. Since clots obstructing an artery supplying blood to the brain cause the majority of strokes, the last thing you need are too many red blood cells. Fortunately, doctors can usually treat this condition with drugs that thin your blood. (See chapter 7.)

Extra red blood cells are more likely to trigger clots.

Mini-Strokes: Public Enemy #4

People who have had mini-strokes called transient ischemic attacks or TIAs (brief episodes of paralysis, slurring of speech and loss of sight that mimic stroke symptoms) are almost ten times more likely to have a stroke than people of the same age and sex who haven't.

In one large study, for example, about 40 percent of those who suffered one or more TIAs went on to have a stroke.

Forty percent of those who have mini-strokes may go on to have a full-fledged stroke.

That's why it's so vitally important to know the physical symptoms that mean you're having a TIA and to seek medical help immediately. Chapter 3 is devoted to understanding TIAs and learning what can be done to treat them and reduce your risk of having a stroke.

High Cholesterol: Public Enemy #5

High levels of blood cholesterol, the fatty substance that travels through your bloodstream, contribute strongly to the development of atheroscle-

rosis—which is the root cause of a majority of
strokes. Cholesterol is also one of the three major
risk factors for heart disease. For both these reasons, you should do everything in your power to
keep your cholesterol at healthy levels. (See the
section, "What Do the Numbers Mean?" on page
36.) If you can slow or prevent the development of
atherosclerosis and heart disease, you're two important steps closer to preventing a stroke.

Keep your cholesterol level down.

Why do high cholesterol levels aid and abet
atherosclerosis? Studies show that this fatty substance joins with other fats and calcium to form
the hardened deposits that narrow your arteries
and indicate that you have the disease.

Cigarettes: Public Enemy #6

Until the last few years, the link between cigarette
smoking and an increased risk of stroke was not
very strong. It seemed to make sense that smoking
would increase the risk of stroke just the way it
increases the risk of heart disease. But researchers
hadn't been able to prove the connection.

Then, late in 1986, researchers from the National Heart, Lung, and Blood Institute and several
other institutions published a landmark study in
the *New England Journal of Medicine,* showing
that male smokers had two to three times the risk
of stroke as nonsmokers. And that was even after
they took into account the men's ages, blood pressure levels, coronary heart disease and other risk
factors. The men were enrolled in the Honolulu
Heart Study, which began following a large group
of men in 1965 to see which of them developed
cardiovascular disease.

Male smokers have two to three times the risk of nonsmokers.

Then, Boston University's Dr. Wolf and several others reported that they also had been able to
find a very definite connection between smoking
and risk of stroke in the Framingham population.
Dr. Wolf, reporting the results of the study in early

Smoke gets in more than your eyes.

1987 at an annual stroke conference sponsored by the AHA, said that male smokers had a 40 percent greater chance of having a stroke than their counterparts who didn't smoke. Female smokers had a 60 percent higher risk of stroke than women who didn't smoke. That excess risk occurred in smokers with or without high blood pressure and other major cardiovascular risk factors. Those who *did* have high blood pressure, of course, simply multiplied their risk even more.

Dr. Wolf and his associates found that while there was an increasing hazard depending on the number of cigarettes smoked, there was also good news for the 50 percent of smokers in Framingham who managed to quit during the study. "After four to five years, the people who stopped smoking had a rate of stroke like that of people who never smoked," says Dr. Wolf. The same happy result was found among the men who took part in the Honolulu Heart Study. Former smokers had only a slight excess risk of stroke when compared with nonsmokers.

You slash your risk of stroke when you quit.

The bottom line? Quitting smoking is worth it. Not only does it quickly reduce your risk of stroke, but studies examining the strong link between heart disease and smoking have found that within one year of quitting, heart attack risk falls by 50 percent. And within ten years, quitters who had smoked a pack a day or less had the same risk of death from heart disease as those who'd never smoked. Since heart disease is such a strong risk factor for stroke, you get a double beneficial effect.

Smoking may trigger clots.

What is it about smoking that aggravates your risk of stroke? Researchers can only speculate at this point, but they think that smoking may trigger the formation of blood clots, which can cause strokes. Smoking tends to thicken the blood by raising the red blood cell count, a major risk factor for stroke. It also increases fibrinogen, a substance which promotes clotting and increases blood viscosity, and makes blood platelets more sticky and likely to aggregate into a clot.

Alcohol: Public Enemy #7

Studies of large populations, such as the Framingham study and the Honolulu Heart Study, have also shown a link between alcohol consumption and stroke. In Framingham, for example, researchers were able to link an increased number of all kinds of strokes to men who drank. And in Honolulu, male drinkers suffered more of the most fatal kind of stroke—the cerebral hemorrhage. Women were not included in these studies for a number of reasons, one of which was that not enough of them in the study populations were admitted drinkers.

Other studies have only strengthened the ties between alcohol and stroke. A second look at the men in the Honolulu Heart Study, for example, showed that the risk of hemorrhagic stroke more than *doubled* for light drinkers and nearly *tripled* for those considered to be heavy drinkers. The risk remained, even after taking into account the men's blood pressure levels. This is important, because some earlier studies had suggested that the reason heavy drinkers suffered more strokes was probably because alcohol raised the blood pressure. The new Honolulu study findings showed that alcohol increased stroke risk independently of blood pressure.

Your risk of stroke triples if you regularly have three or more alcoholic drinks a day.

What is it about alcohol that raises your risk of having a stroke? Studies have shown that alcohol can increase your blood pressure, trigger irregular heartbeats like atrial fibrillation and weaken your heart in other ways. It's also been shown to thicken your blood and cause the arteries leading to your brain to go into spasm, making it harder for nutrient-rich blood to get through. Some doctors also suspect that alcohol contributes to the narrowing of the arteries leading to your brain.

What's a heavy drinker? In the Honolulu study, it was defined as someone who drank the equivalent of three or more drinks a day. Light drinkers consumed the equivalent of about one drink a day.

Alcohol's effect on stroke risk declines as you cut back on drinking.

The good news from this study, however, is that the men who reduced the amount of alcohol they consumed were at a much lower risk of stroke than the men who continued to drink as much or more. This suggests that alcohol may have only a temporary effect on your risk of stroke—one that declines as you cut back on the drinks.

Some doctors in England also looked at alcohol consumption in two similar groups, one of which consisted of people who had recently experienced strokes. Their study found that the risk of stroke was four times higher in heavy drinkers than in nondrinkers. In this study, heavy drinkers were defined as those who drank more than 30 drinks a week. The risk remained, even after the researchers took into account the people's blood pressure and smoking habits.

Teetotalers may not have the lowest risk.

The study also found, however, that light drinkers, defined as those who drank one to ten drinks a week, had a smaller risk of stroke than the teetotalers. Although this makes it look like you're better off if you drink a little, experts in the field were quick to say that the number of people observed to benefit from drinking was statistically too small to lead to the conclusion that light drinking is actually good for you.

Physical Inactivity: Public Enemy #8

Couch potatoes get more of everything—including heart attacks and strokes.

Physical inactivity—less than 4 or 5 hours of weekly exertion—has been linked to an increase in heart disease. And, since people with heart disease are more vulnerable to stroke, it becomes important as a risk factor for stroke. The Framingham study showed that people who were less physically active were at higher risk of suffering from coronary heart disease. Another large study of almost 17,000 Harvard alumni found that avid exercisers had death rates that were one-third lower than their sedentary counterparts.

Becoming more physically active may help you fight other risk factors for stroke, too. Some studies have shown that exercise can help fight hypertension, obesity and diabetes. And exercise has been shown to have a beneficial effect on your cholesterol levels.

Obesity: Public Enemy #9

Excess weight is like physical inactivity—it hasn't been linked independently as a risk factor for stroke, but being overweight can sure increase your chances of having other risk factors for stroke. An increase in your weight, for example, can mean an increase in your blood pressure. Being overweight also contributes to diabetes, heart disease and increased cholesterol levels. A recent look at people in the Framingham Heart Study showed that being overweight was a predictor of who would develop cardiovascular disease.

Extra pounds may mean extra risks.

Diabetes Mellitus: Public Enemy #10

There's no question that having diabetes—excess sugar in your blood—raises your risk of having a stroke. Studies have shown that although both sexes are vulnerable, women are even more so than men.

Although experts generally have believed that what makes diabetes a risk factor for stroke is its strong association with hypertension and heart disease, a study of diabetic men in the Honolulu Heart Study recently revealed that even after those factors were taken into account, diabetics still had a greater risk of stroke. The risk was just about *double* that of nondiabetics.

Diabetes doubles your risk.

Does treating diabetes decrease your risk of stroke? The jury is still out on this one. "We can control blood sugar only imperfectly," says Dr. Wolf. "We can't control sugar metabolism completely, or make it like a nondiabetic's. And be-

sides, the basic metabolism problem that causes
diabetes to occur remains, no matter how it's being
treated."

Nevertheless, it's important to have blood
sugar checked regularly and keep it under the best
control possible if it's excessive. Why? For one
thing, it's been shown that early detection and
treatment of diabetes may reduce your risk of coronary heart disease. Also, the Honolulu study
showed that people with poorly controlled diabetes or diabetes of long duration had an added
risk of stroke.

"The good news for diabetics is that if you
keep diabetes well controlled, it's likely you *can*
reduce your risk of stroke," says Robert D. Abbott,
Ph.D., a biostatistician from the National Heart,
Lung, and Blood Institute, who was the lead author of the Honolulu study.

What is it about diabetes that increases your
risk of stroke? Experts think diabetes may contribute to atherosclerosis, possibly by causing damage
to arteries and allowing them to absorb more fatty
cholesterol deposits. Diabetes may also increase
the thickness of the blood, thus leaving you more
vulnerable to clots.

Keep your blood sugar under control.

Diabetes may help your arteries absorb cholesterol.

Noisy Arteries: Public Enemy #11

A bruit (pronounced *brew-ee*) is an abnormal
sound that your doctor can hear when he places a
stethoscope over an artery. It's usually a signal that
fatty deposits are building up within that artery
due to atherosclerosis. When a doctor hears a bruit
in one of your carotid arteries—the arteries in
your neck—it means your risk of having a stroke
is twice that of someone without the bruit. Unless
you have other symptoms of a pending stroke (like
a transient ischemic attack), however, a carotid
bruit is chiefly just a sign of advancing atherosclerosis. It doesn't necessarily mean that a clot will
form or get stuck in that particular artery and
cause a stroke.

What should you do if your doctor hears this sound? Although doctors disagree on how much you can reverse the damage already done to arteries by atherosclerosis, many believe you can slow it down by changing your diet and exercising in an effort to reduce cholesterol levels.

A carotid bruit is an alarm bell in your arteries.

Who's at Risk?

Your risk of stroke is strongly related to your age. The incidence of stroke doubles in each decade after you turn 55 years old, although almost 30 percent of those who suffer strokes are younger than 65.

Men tend to have a greater risk of stroke than women, especially under age 65. Blacks are also much more susceptible to strokes than whites— their risk is over 60 percent higher. One possible reason for this is that blacks suffer more from hypertension than whites.

If you've already had a stroke, or if you have a family history of strokes, this also puts you at greater risk.

Family always counts.

Studies have also shown that people who live in the southeastern United States are more stroke prone than people in other areas of the country. They also indicate that strokes tend to occur more during periods of extreme hot and cold temperatures. Finally, there's some evidence that strokes are more likely to occur among poor people than among the affluent.

One Plus One Equals Three— or Four

"Risk factors don't stand alone," says Dr. Dyken. "They are all interrelated." When it comes to risk factors—one plus one usually equals more than two. What does that mean? Simply, having multiple risk factors is a lot worse than having just one. Risk factors tend to aggravate each other, as well as

Risk factors don't add up when there's more than one. They multiply.

often being troublesome by themselves. If you smoke and have hypertension, for example, you're much more vulnerable to a stroke than if you just had one or the other.

"And some risk factors that aren't very significant by themselves become very important when combined with others. Although it's still controversial, some studies have shown that if you take oral contraceptives and smoke, for example, your risk of stroke increases—especially if you are over 35, suffer from high blood pressure or have other risk factors for stroke.

The Framingham Five.

Another explosive combination of risk factors could be called the Framingham Five. Researchers there found that the 10 percent of the population in whom one-third to one-half of all strokes occur have a set of five risk factors. These are high blood pressure, high cholesterol, diabetes, an overdevelopment of the left side of the heart—usually detected by an electrocardiogram—and cigarette smoking. "The more they smoked, the higher their blood pressure, cholesterol and sugar levels, and the greater the overdevelopment of their hearts, the more at risk they were," says Dr. Wolf.

How Much at Risk Are You?

Are you at risk?

When it comes to smoking, drinking, eating a healthy diet, exercising and keeping weight down, most of us know where we stand—and where we need to improve. But how do you know if you've developed—or are at risk of developing—some of the most important risk factors for stroke? How do you know if you have high blood pressure or one of the various heart and blood vessel diseases that underlie so many strokes?

To detect many of these conditions, you need a competent health care provider—someone who can give the kind of examination and run the kinds of tests that let you know where you and your body stand.

Chances are that over the years, you've had your blood pressure checked and have had some tests performed when you visited your doctor for a routine checkup or during an illness. But what we're going to detail in the following pages is a comprehensive and far-reaching evaluation, performed by your doctor, that will outline in very clear terms where you're at risk.

This recommended "blueprint for health" was developed by a committee of nationally prominent physicians and preventive health experts for the American Heart Association (AHA). The evaluation, called *Cardiovascular and Risk Factor Evaluation of Healthy American Adults*, suggests regular five-year checkups starting at the age of 20 for all "apparently healthy" adults. (See the table, "A Timetable for Health," on page 42 for a quick rundown on what kinds of tests are recommended, and when.)

You need a "blueprint" for a stroke-free life.

Of course, you may require additional checkups and tests if you have diseases or conditions that warrant it. The checkups, which become more frequent after age 60, are part of a massive effort to prevent all cardiovascular diseases, including coronary heart disease and stroke. The AHA hopes that by asking family doctors to perform these evaluations, millions of people will be helped in recognizing and treating the risk factors for these diseases.

"We have all realized for years that individual physicians are the main way of reaching the greatest number of people to have their risk factors measured and interpreted," says J. Alan Herd, M.D., a member of the committee that developed the evaluation and medical director of the Institute of Preventive Medicine at the Methodist Hospital in Houston. "I can only reach a few thousand people a year here in Houston. That's a small drop in the bucket compared to the millions of people who could be evaluated by their own doctors."

Your family doctor will keep you on track.

But what if your doctor somehow missed seeing the AHA's recommendations? Or what if you simply want to know more about the tests being performed and what they mean to your health? To aid in these efforts, we'll provide a complete rundown on the AHA evaluation, which you can refer to when you sit down with your doctor. If by some chance your doctor hasn't seen the AHA document, he can send for a free copy by writing to your local chapter of the AHA.

At your initial checkup, no matter what your age, your doctor should obtain what are called "baseline" numbers for all the tests performed. Then, when you return for follow-up visits, he will be able to see, for example, whether or not your blood pressure or cholesterol levels have risen.

The first thing the AHA committee advises your doctor to do is take a detailed medical history, asking you questions about any symptoms for heart disease or stroke which you may have felt. In addition, he should note whether you've had any history of diseases and conditions—high blood pressure, for example—that could affect your cardiovascular system.

Next you'll be asked about your *family's* history of heart disease, stroke, hypertension, diabetes, high cholesterol and other diseases that can affect your cardiovascular system. And finally, you'll answer questions about your use of tobacco, alcohol and other drugs and medications, your diet and exercise habits and the level of stress in your life. You'll also be weighed. All of these, obviously, may in some way also affect the health of your cardiovascular system and therefore your potential for having a heart attack or a stroke.

After the medical history, your doctor should perform a complete physical examination of your cardiovascular system, in which he:

- checks your pulse
- measures your blood pressure
- examines your neck arteries for bruits (those abnormal sounds that are usually an indication that the arteries going to your brain are clogged)

You need some baseline numbers.

Your doctor will ask you more questions than a high school math teacher.

You need a complete physical exam.

- listens to your heart for rate, rhythm and other sounds
- examines your eyes, chest, abdomen, arms, legs, hands, feet and nervous system for other clues as to how well your cardiovascular system is operating

During your first exam, you should have a baseline electrocardiogram—sometimes referred to as an ECG or EKG—if you haven't had one before. An electrocardiogram is designed to check your heartbeat for abnormalities.

These various physical examinations are designed to pick up such important stroke risk factors as irregular heart rhythms, the overenlargement of the left side of the heart, a previous silent heart attack and high blood pressure. They'll also give your doctor clues as to whether and how much you are suffering from atherosclerosis, the clogging of the arteries that precedes so many strokes and heart attacks.

The exam will give your doctor some clues about what's going on inside.

Are You at Risk for Stroke?

Ask yourself the following questions. If you answer yes to any of them, you're at risk of having a stroke. Make an appointment with your doctor today for a stroke evaluation.

- Are you over 55?
- Have others in your family had strokes?
- Do you have high blood pressure?
- Do you have high cholesterol?
- Do you smoke?
- Do you have heart disease?
- Do you drink excessively?
- Are you physically inactive?
- Are you overweight?
- Do you have diabetes?

Finally, your doctor will draw blood and have various blood tests performed, especially for cholesterol and blood sugar levels. Many doctors also check your blood in other ways, and these tests could pick up another very important risk factor for stroke, namely an abnormally high red blood cell count.

What Do the Numbers Mean?

Now you know what will happen during your checkup. But what exactly do all those numbers mean? And what do you do once you know you have a risk factor that can be treated? Here's a more detailed look at some of the measurements your doctor will take, most notably your blood pressure, cholesterol levels and blood sugar levels, and what the AHA recommends as a course of action.

Blood pressure. When it comes to blood pressure, you can breathe easiest if your readings are under 140 for systolic pressure (that's the top number) and under 90 for diastolic pressure (the bottom number). These are the numbers for normal blood pressure that the Joint National Committee on Detection, Evaluation and Treatment of High Blood Pressure named in its most recent report. From there, as the numbers go up, there are various kinds of high blood pressure.

> Your blood pressure should be less than 140/90.

If your blood pressure is in the high normal to mildly elevated ranges, your doctor will want to do follow-up readings to recheck it. The good news is that you may not need medication to bring it down to normal again. Watching your salt intake, losing weight and drinking less, along with other lifestyle changes such as exercise, could do the trick.

> Minor changes in your daily regimen can lower your blood pressure.

If your high blood pressure is moderate to severe, your doctor will perform other tests and do follow-up readings and may place you on medication to bring your blood pressure down.

Total cholesterol. The initial cholesterol test your doctor will order for you will measure what's called your total cholesterol. A "good" cholesterol reading is determined depending on your age and sex. (See the table, "Is Your Total Cholesterol Too High?" below for the cholesterol levels that are right for you.)

If your cholesterol is in the desirable area, you probably don't need another cholesterol test for at least five years. If you have other risk factors for cardiovascular disease, however, your doctor may alter that schedule. And despite your low risk, you should be sure to stick to the low-fat, low-cholesterol diet recommended for all Americans. (See chapter 4.) It may prevent your cholesterol levels from rising and retard the development of atherosclerosis.

Get your cholesterol checked.

Is Your Total Cholesterol Too High?

What's a "good" total cholesterol level? Studies have shown that it depends on your age and sex. This table details desirable and high cholesterol levels per milligram for men and women ages 20 and up. If your total cholesterol is between the two numbers for your age and sex, you have a moderate and increasing risk level.

AGE	MEN		WOMEN	
	Desirable (mg/dl)	High (mg/dl)	Desirable (mg/dl)	High (mg/dl)
20–24	<151	>181	<154	>186
25–29	<167	>202	<166	>198
30–34	<180	>215	<166	>199
35–39	<185	>224	<174	>209
40–44	<193	>231	<180	>220
45–49	<200	>237	<191	>231
50–54	<200	>240	<200	>240
55–59	<203	>240	<214	>251
60–64	<204	>240	<211	>251
65–69	<203	>253	<218	>259
70+	<203	>240	<211	>249

SOURCE: Adapted from *Circulation*, June 1987.
NOTE: < = less than; > = more than

A Message to All Americans: Know Your Cholesterol Level

"Know Your Cholesterol Level." It's a slogan that public health advocates say should be as important to us as the one telling us to get our blood pressure checked. The link between high blood cholesterol levels and atherosclerosis, the disease that underlies most strokes and heart attacks, is strong and ominous.

But getting your blood cholesterol levels checked is more complicated than having your blood pressure checked for a couple of reasons. To find out your cholesterol, you need to have blood taken (usually at your doctor's office), sent to a lab and analyzed—with a lag time of one to several days before you learn the results. Blood pressure can be measured and learned on the spot—at public booths or at home with a handy home blood pressure monitor.

And while most doctors know what numbers constitute high blood pressure, many doctors don't have the most up-to-date information on what are safe blood cholesterol levels. So your doctor may tell you not to worry over a cholesterol level that specialists in the field now think *is* worth worrying about. Two recent studies showed that an alarming number of people found to have high-risk blood cholesterol levels were told by their doctors to do nothing.

What's a concerned health care consumer to do? There are several hopeful signs on the horizon. If you're having trouble making the time to get a cholesterol test, look for cholesterol screen-

If your total cholesterol is between desirable and high, you'll want to pay particular attention to other risk factors such as smoking, hypertension, obesity and a family or personal history of coronary heart disease.

Your doctor may also want to order additional cholesterol tests for you to measure certain

ing programs at "health fairs" and the like in your community. They're growing more popular as medical technology is making it easier to analyze blood quickly with special machines that do it on the spot. Then confirm the "quickie" test with one from a lab, to which your doctor can refer you, when you have the time.

If your doctor seems to ignore a blood cholesterol level you've been advised is too high, take heart. (See the table, "Is Your Total Cholesterol Too High?" on page 37 for the most widely accepted numbers.) The National Cholesterol Education Program is making sure that primary care physicians receive lots of up-to-date information on what experts feel are high cholesterol levels. Doctors are also being strongly encouraged to offer meaningful help to people who need to trim their diets of excess fat and dietary cholesterol—the first line of defense against high blood cholesterol levels.

What's meaningful help? It usually means that they coordinate a team of staff members (nurses, physician's assistants and others) to offer you education about how to change your diet. They should also make available the counseling and expertise of registered dietitians if you need help in changing your eating habits.

If your doctor doesn't offer this kind of help, you can contact the National Cholesterol Education Program, National Heart, Lung, and Blood Institute, 4733 Bethesda Avenue, Suite 530, Bethesda, MD 20814. Ask for information on ways to change your diet and then pass on the program's address to your physician.

components of cholesterol called low-density lipoprotein (LDL) cholesterol and high-density lipoprotein (HDL) cholesterol. These will tell your doctor more about your actual risk of developing cardiovascular heart disease.

If your total cholesterol is definitely high, you will need to have additional cholesterol tests after a

Switch to a low-fat, low-cholesterol diet.

12-hour overnight fast to measure HDL, LDL and other components of cholesterol to confirm it. Your efforts to change to a low-fat, low-cholesterol diet will have to be very strenuous. If your cholesterol levels don't respond to changes in your diet, you may need to start taking a cholesterol-lowering drug. But the AHA doesn't recommend these drugs until you've given the diet route a very strong try.

HDL cholesterol. For once, there's something nice you can say about a type of cholesterol. What makes HDL cholesterol the good guy among so many bad? Scientists speculate that HDL cholesterol may act as a kind of vacuum in your arteries, removing harmful cholesterol particles and keeping them from attaching to arterial walls, where they build up and cause clots. Whatever the reason, studies have unquestionably shown that *higher* levels of HDL *decrease* your risk of coronary heart disease. Higher levels protect you. An HDL cholesterol level of 45 mg/dl (milligrams per deciliter) for men and 55 mg/dl for women is considered good.

HDL is the "good" cholesterol.

Another way of evaluating HDL levels is to compare them in a ratio with your total cholesterol figures. Studies have shown that less than a 4.5:1 ratio of total cholesterol to HDL cholesterol is a good one to aim for. What that means, for example, is if your total cholesterol level is 200, your HDL cholesterol should be at least 45.

You can increase HDL levels several ways. Among them: Lose weight if you're fat, exercise more and stop smoking.

LDL cholesterol. If HDL wears the white hat among the different kinds of cholesterol, then LDL wears the black one. *Higher* levels of LDL cholesterol *increase* your risk of heart disease.

LDL is the "bad" cholesterol.

An LDL cholesterol reading gives your doctor even more detailed information on the kinds of cholesterol present in your bloodstream. Doctors often compare LDL and HDL levels, using a risk ratio similar to the one for total cholesterol and

HDL. In this case, an LDL/HDL cholesterol ratio of 2.6:1 is what you should aim for. (See the table, "Is Your LDL Cholesterol Too High?" below to determine what your LDL levels should be.) Like total cholesterol levels, that figure is determined by your age and sex.

Blood sugar. Since diabetes increases your risk of both heart attack and stroke, it's very important that your blood sugar be tested at regular intervals. As we mentioned earlier, detecting and treating diabetes in its early stages may reduce the risk of coronary heart disease, an important risk factor for stroke.

If you're carrying extra weight, have your blood sugar checked every year after you turn 50.

Your blood sugar will be judged high if you have two readings of 140 mg/dl or above. Losing weight and increasing exercise may help reduce your risk. In fact, if you are overweight, your doc-

Is Your LDL Cholesterol Too High?

What's a "good" LDL cholesterol level? It all depends on your age and sex. Here's a list. If your LDL cholesterol is between the two numbers for your age and sex, you have a moderate and increasing risk level.

AGE	MEN		WOMEN	
	Desirable (mg/dl)	High (mg/dl)	Desirable (mg/dl)	High (mg/dl)
20–24	< 95	>118	< 97	>118
25–29	<109	>138	<102	>126
30–34	<117	>144	<103	>129
35–39	<124	>154	<110	>139
40–44	<127	>157	<116	>146
45–49	<132	>163	<120	>150
50–54	<135	>162	<127	>160
55–59	<137	>168	<137	>168
60–64	<132	>165	<141	>168
65–69	<138	>170	<143	>184
70+	<134	>164	<139	>170

SOURCE: Adapted from *Circulation*, June 1987.
NOTE: < = less than; > = more than

A Timetable for Health: The American Heart Association's Recommendations for Periodic Health Examinations

In this table, an "X" indicates this test or medical procedure should occur at this age.

Age	Medical History	Physical Exam	Blood Pressure	Cholesterol	Body Weight	Blood Sugar	ECG	Baseline Chest X-ray
20	X	X	X	X	X	X	X	
25, 30, 35	X	X	X	X	X	X		
40	X	X	X	X	X	X	X	X
45, 50, 55	X	X	X	X	X	X		
60	X	X	X	X	X	X	X	
61–75 (every 2½ years)	X	X	X	optional*	X	X		
75+ (every year)	X	X	X	optional*	X	optional*		

SOURCE: The American Heart Association.

NOTE: Blood pressure should be taken every 2½ years in normal patients.

*If baseline levels are well documented.

tor may order blood sugar tests more frequently. The AHA recommends that people who are mildly overweight have it tested twice as often as people of normal weight after age 45. If you are really obese, your blood sugar should be measured every year after you turn 50.

Additional tests. If you smoke, be prepared to undergo additional tests that include an evaluation of your lung function and a chest x-ray. Your doctor may also suggest more frequent cardiovascular exams and electrocardiogram tests as well.

Now that you're finished at your doctor's office, you know exactly where you stand in terms of risk for stroke. The rest of this book is dedicated to helping you learn how to change the risks you can through positive lifestyle change.

Get a lung function test if you smoke.

Chapter 3

Warning: Mini-Strokes Mean the Threat Is Real

Mini-strokes, or *transient ischemic attacks* (TIAs) as they're known in medical lingo, are the most vivid warning signals your body uses to tell you that you're on the road to a major stroke. They consist of any one or a combination of the following strokelike symptoms, which usually come and go over a short period of time.

- You suddenly feel weak or numb in your face, arm, hand or leg.
- You lose the ability to speak clearly or have trouble understanding the speech of others.
- You experience a dimness or loss of vision—commonly only in one eye.
- You feel dizzy or unsteady or you suddenly fall, and you can't attribute it to any particular cause.

If you suspect you've had a mini-stroke, you should seek medical help immediately. A TIA

Most TIAs last 8 to 14 minutes.

mimics what a real stroke would do to your ability to speak, comprehend, see or even use an arm or a leg. The major difference is that with a TIA, the symptoms usually go away rapidly—more than half last less than 8 to 14 minutes and 90 percent last less than 2 to 6 hours (that's why they're called "transient" attacks). In a small number of cases, TIA symptoms can last longer—but never more than 24 hours.

Short or long, TIAs are powerful omens. As many as 20 to 40 percent of those who have them go on to suffer full-blown strokes. People who've had one or more mini-strokes, in fact, are almost ten times more likely to have a stroke than people of the same age and sex who are TIA-free.

Twenty to 40 percent of those who experience TIAs will have strokes within a week.

And if a stroke is to occur, chances are good that it'll come soon. "The greatest risk is in the first week after a TIA happens," says Harold P. Adams, Jr., M.D., a professor of neurology and director of the Cerebrovascular Diseases Division at the University of Iowa. That's why it's so critical that you receive medical attention immediately after you suspect you've had a TIA.

But if after reading our detailed description of the symptoms, you realize that—sometime in the past—you may have had a TIA, you should still see your doctor right away. Studies show that some people can go as long as five years after a TIA before they eventually have a stroke. So don't feel as though you're out of the woods if your suspected TIA occurred a while ago.

But why do TIAs occur? Doctors suspect that in most cases, it's because a blood clot has gotten stuck in one of the arteries supplying blood to your

A blood clot gets stuck—then breaks free.

brain. Mercifully, the clot breaks free and dissolves, and soon your brain is once again receiving its life-sustaining supply of oxygen and other nutrients. Your stroke symptoms disappear, leaving no lasting damage.

As you might suspect, this logjam is more likely to originate in arteries that are damaged due to atherosclerosis, high blood pressure and other diseases. The clots tend to form at damaged points in your arteries. It's there that atherosclerotic fatty deposits—made up of cholesterol and other arterial debris—have narrowed your arteries to the point where it's hard for blood to get through.

Blood clots can form logjams in your arteries.

Clots can develop right in damaged arteries as a response to that damage. These clots can break loose and lodge at points where the artery narrows, or can come there after forming in a diseased heart. And if it happens once, it can happen again. But next time, it could stay lodged and trigger a full-blown stroke.

Another theory about why TIAs happen is that when an artery becomes completely clogged, your body does a miraculous thing: It sends blood to your brain via other blood supply routes that immediately form to do the job. Hence, your strokelike TIA symptoms disappear once your brain begins to get nourishment from these alternative supply routes.

Your body can save you.

You shouldn't feel complacent, however, just because your body has saved you this time. Even if your brain is getting blood from other arteries, the fact remains that an artery is either significantly narrowed or completely shut down. That still leaves you in great danger of a stroke. If you've had a TIA, you may feel rather like a driver who's just missed crashing broadside into another car in traffic—frightened by how close you came to total devastation.

Now let's look at the symptoms of TIA in detail, and then at what doctors can do about them.

Hands That Don't Work

Mamie couldn't explain it, but something was wrong with her right hand. It just wasn't working right. When she was turning her key in the door to go into the house, it was as though she'd lost the ability to manipulate her fingers to do that simple task. Her right arm felt heavy, too, and when she touched it, it seemed to have lost feeling. "I must have spent too much time at my computer terminal today," she thought.

Mamie smiled weakly at her husband, John, as he came into the room, but he laughed uneasily and asked her why she was greeting him with such a lopsided grin. Mamie reached up to touch the right side of her face and realized that it, too, had lost feeling—as though she'd had a Novocain injection at the dentist. "John," she said, suddenly feeling like the room was spinning around, "I'm going to faint!"

A lopsided smile.

What Mamie was feeling were some of the most frightening symptoms of a TIA or a stroke—the dizziness and loss of feeling in one side of her body. In Mamie's case, her symptoms had subsided by the time she and her husband reached the hospital emergency room—which led her doctor to believe she'd had a TIA instead of a stroke.

But you don't have to have all of Mamie's symptoms to have experienced a mini-stroke. "You can feel weak or numb in just your hand, or just your face, or any combination of body parts on one side," says Dr. Adams. And although it's very rare to have an entire side of your body affected, you might also have a tingling sensation in whatever part is affected.

Weakness or numbness in any part of your body can indicate a TIA.

Your leg can also feel numb, says Dr. Adams, although that's less often a symptom. What does "numb" feel like? "The leg would feel heavy," Dr. Adams replies. "You'd feel as though you were dragging it. And you'd be unsteady on your feet."

A Mouthful of Mashed Potatoes

Across town from where Mamie lived, a man named George was having an argument with his wife, Jane. Suddenly she noticed that he was speaking strangely. "George," she said, "what's the matter? You're not making any sense." He sounded tired and confused—like he was losing his mind.

What frightened George was that he could hear his wife talking, but suddenly the words she was saying didn't make sense to him either.

Jane bolted from the table and called her daughter, who lived nearby. "Honey, come over right away. Your dad's very sick." But by the time Jane returned to the table, George's speech seemed to be back to normal. And he was making sense again.

"George, what happened?" she asked in relief. "I couldn't understand you there for a minute." Equally relieved, George smiled at his wife and said, "That's okay, I couldn't understand you either—but now I can."

George had experienced another symptom of both TIAs and stroke: a loss of the ability to communicate properly or understand speech. "This is a hard symptom for a victim to spot," says Dr. Adams. "It's most often noticed by observers."

Someone who's experiencing a TIA can also experience a slurring of speech that's brought on by a weakening of the facial muscles. "It would sound a lot like you were trying to talk with mashed potatoes in your mouth," says Dr. Adams. In this case, the words you say make sense, it's just that you slur them as they come out.

Temporary speech problems can also signal a TIA.

People around you are more likely to notice a speech problem than you are.

A TIA Fog

Tom was lining up at the dock after an enjoyable day out fishing on his boat when suddenly he felt his vision dimming in one eye. "It was like a fog had settled over my eye, sort of the way it can suddenly come in when you're out on the water," he later told his doctor, using an image familiar to most fishermen. "Or like a curtain or shade had been drawn over my eye."

Tom quickly asked his son to take over the wheel as his eyesight continued to worsen. Feeling definitely unsteady on his feet, he sat down. Then, suddenly, the "fog" lifted and Tom could see per-

A fisherman who couldn't see.

fectly again. His son insisted on steering the boat the rest of the way in, and he strongly urged his father to see a doctor—right away.

Partial or complete blindness, which commonly strikes in one eye but can affect both, is another common symptom of a TIA, says Dr. Adams. When it affects both eyes, it's like your eyesight becomes blurred or out of focus. "In a few cases," he explains, "your vision can go down to a pin in the center, sort of like a camera. Or it can look as though you're seeing sparkles, stars or lightning bolts in front of your eyes. Occasionally a patient will also complain of double vision, but that's not very common."

Any distortion of your vision can indicate a TIA.

You might also notice that you suddenly can't see out of one side of your eye, adds Roger E. Kelley, M.D., director of the Clinical Stroke Service at the University of Miami's School of Medicine. "In fact, your vision could be cut off in half of both eyes," says Martin Reivich, M.D., a University of Pennsylvania professor of neurology. "Sometimes it's hard for patients to tell whether they're completely blind in the left eye, for example, or have just lost their vision in the left half of each eye."

Unexpected Dizziness or Unsteadiness

Dizziness or unsteadiness, such as the kind experienced by both Tom and Mamie, is rarely in and of itself the sign of a TIA. But when it accompanies other TIA symptoms, like loss of eyesight or weakness and numbness, it can be an added sign that something is wrong. "Here we're not talking about occasional dizziness when you get out of bed or up from a chair," says Dr. Adams, "but real vertigo— like you're on a merry-go-round." Actually, you should always report any dizziness to your physician. Dizziness is a symptom of many diseases besides stroke and TIA and should be checked.

Dizziness can indicate a TIA when it's accompanied by other symptoms.

Checking It All Out

Mamie and her husband, George and his wife and daughter, and Tom and his son all wound up that night at the emergency room of the local community hospital. While anxious relatives waited, doctors began a series of tests and procedures designed to tell them exactly what had happened and whether the symptoms they'd experienced were TIAs or some other problems. (See the box, "Brain Tumor or TIA?" below.)

Finding out what happened.

All three did the right thing in getting medical help right away, according to doctors who treat patients with TIAs and strokes. "You don't know if the attack you had was going to be transient—or whether in the next hour you might have a real stroke," says Dr. Reivich. And Dr. Adams agrees.

TIAs are real emergencies. Don't ignore them.

Brain Tumor or TIA?

If you experience numbness or weakness in any part of your body, a loss of speech or vision or other symptoms of a TIA, you might rightly suspect that these are warnings of a possible stroke and head for your nearest hospital.

And that's exactly what you should be doing. But you may be suffering from an entirely different disease altogether. Here's just a partial list of some of the other diseases of which your symptoms might be a warning.

- Brain tumor
- Carpal tunnel syndrome (a pinched nerve in your wrist, which can cause numbness and tingling in your hands)
- Eye disease (including glaucoma)
- Inner ear or Ménière's disease
- Low blood sugar
- Migraine headaches

"These attacks are true emergencies. You need to be seen by a doctor."

When Mamie, George and Tom were admitted, the hospital staff carefully checked all three. Their temperatures and blood pressures were taken and they had blood drawn for testing. The blood tests that are routinely performed for people suspected of having TIAs check the thickness of the blood and the amount of cholesterol and sugar that it contains—all three tests could give doctors clues about what possibly caused the TIA.

Doctors at the hospital also performed electrocardiograms to check for such things as a silent heart attack or irregular heartbeats, which can cause clots to form and travel to the arteries supplying your brain. Doctors also know that a great many people who show signs of stroke are at risk of having heart attacks, so they want to prevent coronary problems, too.

While carefully questioning the three about the TIA symptoms they'd experienced, their doctors also listened to their carotid arteries—the arteries in the neck—to detect abnormal sounds which signal that fatty deposits have built up there and may cause TIAs.

There are also several other, more complex, tests that patients like Mamie, George and Tom would be likely to undergo, depending on their individual medical condition, their age and their overall health. Here's a rundown.

CT scan. This test's long name is *computerized tomography,* and it's performed on virtually all patients with suspected TIAs. The CT scan uses a computer to construct black-and-white pictures of the brain generated by multiple x-rays beamed through the head.

It can be performed as soon as a TIA patient arrives at the hospital to give doctors quick information on whether the brain has been damaged by the symptoms described. It also lets doctors

A peek into your brain.

know for sure that your TIA isn't something else—like a brain tumor. CT scans also enable doctors to see if there's any bleeding or if your brain has sustained any damage from "silent strokes" in the past.

MRI. This test, whose full name is *magnetic resonance imaging,* is similar to a CT scan in what it detects, except that it's even more sensitive and requires no radiation from x-rays. It uses a magnetic field to gives doctors detailed pictures of your brain so they can determine if there's any damage. A more recently developed test, MRI will one day replace CT scans as the test of choice for examining the structure of the brain, says Dr. Reivich.

MRI produces detailed pictures.

PET scan. *Positron emission tomography* is still being used only experimentally at university hospitals, but doctors have high hopes that one day it may be available for use everywhere. While a CT scan or MRI shows how your brain looks, a PET scan also shows how your brain is working—how it's using oxygen, glucose and the other nutrients it needs to operate.

A recent study at the University of Pennsylvania showed that while a CT scan can locate only brain cells that have died, a PET scan can locate brain cells that have been weakened and damaged. It does this by identifying which cells are absorbing the most glucose—the active, healthy ones—and which are absorbing very little—the weakened, damaged ones.

PET scans can even detect weakened brain cells.

"We're now performing a new study to see if PET could help us in identifying which TIA patients have the most weakened and damaged brain cells and thus may derive the greatest benefit from surgery to get blood flowing properly again," says Dr. Reivich. The researchers have already found, for example, that some TIA patients' brain cells that look normal and healthy suddenly start to look weak when they're asked to do something as simple as allowing the patient to talk. Thus, the

PET scan can give your doctor a lot of information about your brain to guide him into making a decision about how to treat you.

Ultrasound scan. While doctors are very concerned about how your brain is operating after you come in with the symptoms of a TIA, they also want to find out why you may have had the TIA in the first place. Since most TIAs occur because arteries supplying the brain are clogged and damaged, one of a physician's chief goals is to identify the artery that is causing the problem, the location of damage and the degree of blockage. He may begin that search by using an ultrasound scanner, which creates pictures based on high-frequency sound to detect obstructions in the neck arteries that supply your brain with blood. An attachment to the ultrasound scanner, called a Doppler, can enable physicians to actually hear abnormalities of flow in your artery while seeing them on the screen.

Ultrasound scans can detect any obstruction.

The advantage of using an ultrasound scan is that it's noninvasive, that is, it looks at your arteries from outside your body. It's always less risky to do that than to enter your body, as some artery tests must. But the disadvantage of ultrasound scans—and other noninvasive tests that check your arteries—is that, although quite sensitive, they generally don't give as accurate a picture of the potential damage inside your arteries as an invasive test. Nevertheless, these tests are widely used, especially as a complement and follow-up to invasive tests such as the arteriogram.

Ultrasound helps look at your arteries.

Arteriogram. An arteriogram is a series of x-ray pictures that show the flow of blood in your arteries. The pictures are taken after dye is injected into a tube which has been inserted into an arm or leg artery and threaded up into your neck arteries. The dye helps doctors see the movement of blood through your brain's arteries and identify blockages. It also helps them decide whether or not you need surgery to repair any damage.

Arteriograms trace your flow of blood.

If you're elderly, in poor health and at high risk of having a stroke, however, doctors may stop short of performing an arteriogram because there's a very small risk that the procedure itself could trigger a stroke. In your case, the doctor may rely on information obtained from noninvasive tests and use various medications to treat you.

Some doctors also feel that if your case is not too severe, you don't need to be considered for surgery and therefore don't need an arteriogram. In fact, this is the most hotly debated subject among doctors who treat patients at risk for stroke. When should a patient be operated on to prevent stroke? When should he be treated with medication? We'll discuss that debate in chapters 7 and 8, which are all about the drugs and surgical techniques being used today to prevent strokes.

For now, let's move on to the changes you yourself can make in your diet, exercise, smoking and drinking habits to ensure that you won't end up in an emergency room like Mamie, George and Tom.

Part **2**

How You Can Prevent a Stroke

Chapter 4

A Food-Lover's Guide to Stroke Prevention

What's eating got to do with your risk of having a stroke? In a word—everything. Many of the staple foods in our current American diet, when eaten to excess, have been fingered in the development of atherosclerosis, heart disease, hypertension, high blood cholesterol, diabetes and—of course—obesity. Sound like a familiar litany of diseases? It should, for they all conspire to put you at risk of having a stroke.

Fortunately, there's an equally large and varied litany of foods that actually reduce your risk of developing any of these diseases, including stroke. But, first let's talk about the foods that put you at risk.

The case against fat, for example, is enormous. Countless studies have now proven that high-fat foods play a key role in raising the amount of cholesterol in your blood. And it's high levels of blood cholesterol that practically make it your des-

The case against fat.

tiny to develop atherosclerosis, the disease that clogs the arteries supplying blood to your brain and heart, and causes most strokes and heart attacks.

Several kinds of studies helped scientists prove that fatty foods are among the chief villains in the high cholesterol/atherosclerosis story. First, when researchers compared large populations of people such as the Japanese, who eat a low-fat diet, with Americans and others who eat a high-fat diet, the Japanese had much lower cholesterol levels and less atherosclerosis. But when Japanese people move to a place like the United States and start eating a high-fat diet, their blood cholesterol starts to rise—along with their risk of developing atherosclerosis.

Evidence from the lab.

Studies of the arteries of animals confirmed what the population studies suggested. They showed that when animals are fed a high-fat diet, their blood cholesterol levels rise and their arteries become narrowed and clogged by atherosclerotic plaque. When a low-fat diet is substituted for a high-fat one, however, those same arteries are cleared of some of the fatty deposits that cause the disease.

A low-fat diet can unclog arteries.

Now studies in people are beginning to confirm what the animal studies showed—that low-fat eating can help fight atherosclerosis. A recent study sponsored by the National Heart, Lung, and Blood Institute, for example, took x-ray pictures of the arteries of a group of men who had severe atherosclerosis. Then they got half of the men to eat low-fat foods and take cholesterol-lowering drugs. The other half went on a low-fat diet but took a placebo (an inactive drug look-alike). After two years, the researchers looked at the men's arteries again and found that not only had the atherosclerosis slowed in the group that ate low-fat foods, in some cases their arteries were *less* clogged than they'd been before.

This was the first study to actually look at people's arteries and see this miraculous effect.

And even though more men in the diet-plus-drug group enjoyed these changes, a respectable 37 percent of the men on diets alone saw their atherosclerosis stop, while another 2.4 percent saw it reverse.

"Clearly, diet had an effect," says David H. Blankenhorn, M.D., chief investigator of the study. "We can infer from our study that if people with atherosclerosis eat a low-fat, low-cholesterol diet (and don't smoke or have high blood pressure), at least 39 percent of them will have stable lesions, that is, their atherosclerosis damage will either diminish or stop progressing."

William Castelli, M.D., director of the renowned Framingham Heart Study, believes that this study and others from around the world suggest that atherosclerosis can be slowed simply by lowering blood cholesterol. "Even more," adds Dr. Castelli, "I think that in some people, diet alone can lower cholesterol enough to reverse the lesions of atherosclerosis."

All these studies have led experts to conclude that for most of us who have higher than normal blood cholesterol levels, reducing the amount of high-fat food we eat is the best first step toward lowering those levels and preventing or reversing atherosclerosis. That's why a major government project, the National Cholesterol Education Program, brought together experts from all over the country for a nationwide campaign to get us all on the path toward a lower-fat eating style—even those of us who currently have healthy blood cholesterol levels.

But giving your arteries a break isn't the only reason to reduce the amount of high-fat food you eat. It can also bring down your blood pressure, according to a growing number of studies. And since high blood pressure is the *number one* risk factor for stroke, that's good news.

Researchers have compared the foods eaten by people in different countries and have found that the Finns, for example, have much higher blood pressure than the Italians. Why? Finns generally

Diet halted atherosclerosis in its tracks.

Putting the nation on a diet.

A low-fat diet can also bring down your blood pressure.

eat a high-fat diet, researchers report. Italians don't. Fortunately, when Finnish people with high blood pressure are put on lower-fat diets, their pressure comes down.

Americans enjoyed a similar effect in a study done by the U.S. Department of Agriculture/Agricultural Research Service Western Human Nutrition Research Center. In that study, even people with normal blood pressure enjoyed a drop in their pressure levels after eating lower-fat foods for just three months, and this translates into a drop in their stroke risk.

Researchers aren't sure yet why eating less fat may help your blood pressure, but some theorize that it may be because your body gets rid of more salt when you eat less fat. And salt can be a powerful blood pressure aggravator.

Do your kidneys a favor.

How does salt contribute to high blood pressure? When your body is carrying around too much salt, your kidneys are in charge of getting rid of it. But one way the kidneys do this is by releasing hormones that raise blood pressure. Moreover, studies of cultures around the world have confirmed salt's role as a chief culprit in raising blood pressure. In countries where little salt is consumed, very few people suffer from high blood pressure. But in a country like the United States, where we eat lots of salt, high blood pressure is rampant.

The High Cost of High Calories

Cutting out the fat usually means cutting calories, too.

If you're overweight, cutting back on calories is just as important as cutting back on fat in a stroke-prevention diet. Luckily, when you trim the fat from your diet, you usually trim calories, too. And if you cut back on some highly sugared foods at the same time, you'll be doing your body a double favor. Not only do sugar's empty calories contribute to weight gain, but a lot of highly sugared foods are also high-fat foods—like ice cream, pie and cake.

Why does being overweight make you stroke-prone? Let's count the ways. For starters, being overweight means you're at greater risk of developing all kinds of cardiovascular diseases, including stroke and heart attack, according to a recent look at overweight people in the Framingham study. And that's regardless of whether you have other cardiovascular risk factors, such as high blood pressure, high blood cholesterol or diabetes.

But these other risk factors are often aggravated by being overweight, too. National surveys of a cross section of Americans found that people who are overweight are nearly *three* times as likely to have high blood pressure than others of normal weight. They're twice as likely to have extremely high blood cholesterol levels. And extra weight also means a three times greater chance of developing diabetes.

Extra weight means extra trouble.

But it does work both ways—as people lose weight, their blood pressure comes back down, according to a subcommittee report of the Joint National Committee on Detection, Evaluation and Treatment of High Blood Pressure prepared on nondrug ways to control high blood pressure. One fascinating way researchers first discovered this, for example, was by noticing that the blood pressures of the people of Leningrad fell while they were besieged and near starvation during World War II. When the siege was lifted and food became available, blood pressures rose again, as did the number of people with high blood pressure.

One final note on being too fat: Studies in recent years have shown that it isn't just the fact that you're overweight—it's where the fat is on your body—that predicts your risk of stroke and heart disease and even possibly hypertension. Swedish researchers have conducted a series of studies showing that people whose fat settles in a potbelly or paunch are at much greater risk than people whose fat shows up on their arms, legs or bottom. If you fit this description, you'll want to make an extra effort to reduce risk factors for

Where's the fat?

Are You Overweight?

How overweight do you have to be before those extra pounds start to threaten your health? The Framingham Heart Study found that people who were heavier than the desirable weights listed below ran a greater risk of developing cardiovascular diseases, including stroke and heart attack. And the risk increased as these people got heavier. For strokes in particular, overweight women were at risk more than men. Women younger than 70, for example, who were 30 percent or more over the desirable weights listed below had *four* times the stroke rate of the leanest group. The Framingham researchers based these weights on information from the 1959 version of the Metropolitan Life Insurance Company's ideal weight charts.

	WOMEN		**MEN**	
Height	**Desirable Weight* (lb.)**	**Height**	**Desirable Weight* (lb.)**	
4'7"	94	5'0"	116	
4'8"	97	5'1"	119	
4'9"	100	5'2"	122	
4'10"	103	5'3"	125	
4'11"	106	5'4"	128	
5'0"	109	5'5"	131	
5'1"	112	5'6"	135	
5'2"	116	5'7"	140	
5'3"	120	5'8"	144	
5'4"	124	5'9"	148	
5'5"	128	5'10"	152	
5'6"	132	5'11"	157	
5'7"	136	6'0"	161	
5'8"	140	6'1"	166	
		6'2"	170	

Source: Adapted from *Circulation*, May 1983.

*Adjusted for shoes and clothing.

An extra 10 percent of body weight can increase your risk of cardiovascular disease.

stroke, including being overweight.

How, exactly, is overweight defined? According to the Framingham statistics, people who were more than 10 percent over their desirable body weights (based on figures from the 1959 version of the Metropolitan Life Insurance Company's Desirable Weight Tables), had an increased risk of developing cardiovascular disease. (See the table, "Are

You Overweight?" on page 62 for a look at those desirable weights.)

So far, we've talked about what you'll want to cut back on among the foods you presently eat. Now we'll list some of the kinds of foods medical evidence has most recently linked with a reduction in atherosclerosis—the process underlying strokes, heart disease and the related risk factors for these diseases. Along with their disease-preventing aspects, these kinds of foods are also naturally low in calories, fat, sugar and salt.

The Stroke Busters

It was the most puzzling paradox scientists had come upon in a long time. Despite the fact that Eskimos ate a diet tremendously high in fatty fish, they had almost no heart disease. Why were the Eskimos spared, when the rest of us eating high-fat foods were turning into stroke-prone butterballs?

A lesson from the Eskimos: Fish offers double protection.

Researchers soon discovered that fish were rich in omega-3 fatty acids, an apparently "good" kind of fat that actually reduces cholesterol and other harmful fats in your blood.

But omega-3's sterling qualities don't stop there. Besides keeping arteries cleaner, omega-3 fatty acids also keep your blood from getting sticky. That reduces the risk of blood clots forming in the arteries. Since so many strokes and heart attacks are triggered by a clot getting stuck in a clogged artery, omega-3 fatty acids offer double protection to people intent on preventing cardiovascular diseases.

But foods high in fiber should also take center stage in your new way of eating. We're talking here about whole grain cereals, bread and pasta; fruits and vegetables; and beans and lentils.

High-fiber foods have become famous for various reasons, including their reputation for fighting constipation and colon cancer. But studies are now showing that the kind of fiber in fruits, vegetables, beans and oat bran can also lower cholesterol and help control blood sugar. So high-fiber

Fiber can lower your cholesterol.

foods play a major role in stroke prevention, too.

An added benefit is that people who start eating high-fiber foods lose weight more easily—probably because they feel fuller and because most high-fiber foods are naturally low in fat. They also tend to be high in carbohydrates, which is the food component you'll be using to fill in for some of the fat you take off your menus.

The most important part of your stroke-busting diet, however, may be fruits and vegetables.

The Stroke Busters: Fruits and Vegetables Rich in Potassium

Fruits and vegetables provide direct and powerful protection against strokes, according to a recent study. Researchers think the mineral potassium, found in so many fruits and vegetables, may be the hero. Here's a list of the richest sources.

Very Good Sources		Good Sources	
Fruits	**Vegetables**	**Fruits**	**Vegetables**
Apple juice	Artichokes	Apples	Asparagus
Bananas	Bamboo shoots	Apricots, dried	Bean sprouts
Blackberries	Beets	Blueberries	Cabbage
Cantaloupe	Beet greens	Cherries	Cauliflower
Grapefruit juice	Broccoli	Grapefruit	Celery
Honeydew melon	Brussels sprouts	Grapes	Corn
Nectarines	Carrots	Pineapple	Eggplant
Orange juice	Collard greens	Pineapple juice	Green beans
Oranges	Lima beans	Plums	Green peppers
Peaches	Parsnips	Tangerines	Lettuce
Pears	Potatoes	—	Mushrooms
Prune juice	Pumpkins	—	Mustard greens
Prunes, dried	Rutabaga	—	Okra
Raisins	Spinach	—	Peas
Strawberries	Split peas	—	Radishes
Watermelon	Winter squash	—	Summer squash
—	Sweet potatoes	—	Turnip greens
—	Tomato juice	—	Zucchini
—	Tomatoes	—	—

SOURCE: Adapted from *Grocery Guide: Tips on Wise Food Selection*, by the American Heart Association.

That's because fruits and vegetables don't just lower your blood sugar and cholesterol. They may also provide direct and powerful protection against strokes, according to a recent study.

How? Scientists aren't sure. But after following 859 people over 12 years, researchers found that those who ate just one extra serving of fresh fruits and vegetables had a 40 percent lower risk of dying from stroke. And the *more* fruits and vegetables people ate, the researchers report, the *less* likely their risk of stroke.

An extra serving of fresh fruits and vegetables each day can reduce your risk of a death due to stroke by 40 percent.

The mineral potassium, found in most fruits and vegetables, appears to be the hero—just as it is for high blood pressure. (See the table, "The Stroke Busters: Fruits and Vegetables Rich in Potassium," on page 64.) As a result, the researchers concluded in the *New England Journal of Medicine,* "These findings support the hypothesis that a high intake of potassium from food sources may protect against stroke-associated deaths."

How to Change the Way You Eat

How many times have you zealously decided to make some positive lifestyle change, like exercising more or eating less, only to find yourself back to your old habits in a few short weeks? Chances are you tried to do too much too soon, and your body, mind and heart rebelled. That's because after a lifetime of doing things a certain way, it's almost impossible to introduce radical change overnight.

Taming the body rebellion.

Don't expect it to be any different when you decide to change your eating habits to prevent a stroke. Your taste preferences for certain foods have been with you probably since you were a child, says Jeannie C. Sykes, Ph.D., a Greensboro, North Carolina, registered dietitian and nutrition consultant who—as president of Creative Health Strategies—is involved in educational projects all over the country that encourage people to make healthy eating changes.

"Most of us learn our taste preferences from our parents," says Dr. Sykes. "We like the foods we eat because of our early exposure to them. And we tend to distrust and dislike foods that are unfamiliar."

But our preferences for certain foods are more adaptable than we think, emphasizes Dr. Sykes. "Think of changes many people have made already. Those who learn to enjoy black coffee, for example, don't understand how they ever drank it with cream and sugar."

Your taste buds are more adaptable than you think.

Many studies on salt preference prove her point, says Dr. Sykes. One study at the University of Pennsylvania, for example, showed that after five months on a low-salt diet, the people involved actually *preferred* soup and crackers with much less salt than they had before starting the diet.

But even though studies show that you can alter your taste preferences, no one is suggesting that you do it quickly. Because it just doesn't work.

A sneak attack on the way you eat.

Sonja L. Connor, a registered dietitian and assistant professor at Oregon Health Sciences University, is the pioneer who came up with the idea of changing the way you eat permanently by making the changes slowly and in phases. Her ideas grew out of the frustration she felt when patients she was trying to help kept slipping back to their old eating habits.

She and her colleagues were trying to encourage people to adopt an eating style designed to prevent strokes and heart disease. "We'd get very negative reactions to the changes we were suggesting," says Connor. "So my colleagues and I decided to try and figure out how we ourselves had managed to make the changes we were now asking others to make. We also observed successful patients—those who had made permanent changes.

"What we found out was that all of us had done it in a slow, gradual way," she says.

Connor, who says her own eating habits used to be like the typical American's, reports that she and her family made their biggest changes toward foods that help prevent stroke and heart disease over *a five-year period*—not an instant makeover by anyone's estimation. "And we're still making changes today," the nutritionist says. "It's a constant process."

Connor and her husband, William E. Connor, M.D., a distinguished heart researcher, decided to launch a study at the Oregon Health Sciences University to find out how much people will change to new ways of eating when the changes are introduced gradually and involve food which will satsify them.

Give yourself time.

The Family Heart Study, as it was called, randomly selected 233 families to participate. At the end of five years, 90 percent of the families were still participating and most had made progress in their quest toward a healthier diet, report the Connors in their book, *The New American Diet.* That's an amazing statistic when you consider that many more people than that usually drop out of such studies.

A 90-percent success rate.

What were the Connors's secrets? They encouraged people to go slowly and change only as much as they felt comfortable with at any given moment. Second, they introduced new foods and new ways of preparing food in attractive, delicious recipes. They realized that no one is going to change to a way of eating that doesn't taste good. And finally, they got whole families involved, recognizing that if permanent change was going to come about, it had to have the support of everyone who lived in the household.

The secret is food that looks and tastes good—and a family that's with you all the way.

How do these guidelines translate into practical tips? Let's use milk as an example. You want to move from using whole milk toward using low-fat milk so you can reduce the saturated fat in your diet. Instead of starting with skim milk, which you and/or your family might balk at, you start with 2 percent milk. Although your family still protests, you demonstrate how little flavor or texture change occurs by using the 2 percent milk in recipes like pancakes.

Once you and your family realize that a recipe

can still taste delicious using lower-fat milk, you've won half the battle. You've won the other half when you can serve the 2 percent milk at the table. But remember, slow change is more likely to become permanent change. So if you don't like the taste of 2 percent milk at first, try using it half and half with whole milk.

Make your changes one at a time.

Another important thing to remember when you're trying to make lifetime changes in your diet is to not tackle too many things all at once. "If you drink a lot of milk," says Dr. Sykes, "that's a huge project all in itself. Work just on that for awhile."

The idea isn't to turn around tomorrow and completely overhaul your whole way of eating. Gradually switch from butter to margarine, or high-fat to lower-fat cheeses, advises Dr. Sykes. Work on things one at a time. And don't tell yourself things like, "I will never eat my favorite food the way I like it again."

Eventually, you won't even think of how you used to eat.

It's too hard for most people to deal with the word *never*, says Dr. Sykes. "If you're working on a food that's a daily part of your diet, you might even try having it the old way once a week or so. Soon you'll probably find you aren't even bothering to do it the old way."

Nutritionists like Dr. Sykes and those who worked on the Family Heart Study are helping people all over the country change their diets in ways such as these. So are experts from the National Heart, Lung, and Blood Institute and the American Heart Association (AHA), both groups devoted to preventing strokes, heart attacks and the diseases that cause them. And in the pages that follow, we'll be giving you their countless tips on how you can do the same, after consulting, of course, with your family doctor. Let's start with cutting back on fat.

The Many Faces of Fat

A fat is a fat is a fat, right? Wrong. There are different kinds of fat—some more benign than others. And although your general goal should be to cut back on all kinds of fat in your diet, it helps to know the good and the bad from the ugly.

In the ugly category, your biggest enemy in the fight against atherosclerosis is *saturated fat,* a fat that's largely found in animal foods, such as meat and dairy products, and a few vegetable oils, most notably coconut and palm oil. You can tell you're dealing with a food high in saturated fat if the fat hardens at room temperature. It's saturated fat that tends to raise your blood cholesterol levels, which leads to the development of atherosclerosis.

Saturated fat's nasty sidekick is *dietary cholesterol,* a steroid alcohol found in animal fats and oils. Dietary cholesterol also raises blood cholesterol levels, especially when it's coupled with a high saturated fat intake. But don't make the mistake of thinking that dietary cholesterol is somehow more important than saturated fat as a blood cholesterol aggravator. It isn't. And even though it seems to make sense, it's dangerous to accord more importance to one than the other.

You may be virtuously avoiding foods high in cholesterol but still eating foods high in saturated fat. Many commercially prepared crackers and baked goods, for example, contain coconut or palm oil. Since those two are nonanimal fats, they contain no cholesterol. But they have nearly *twice* the saturated fat of beef.

A third, more benign form of fat is called *polyunsaturated fat.* It's found in greatest concentrations in vegetable oils, like safflower, sunflower, corn and soybean. You can tell you're dealing with a highly polyunsaturated fat when it stays liquid at room temperature. Polyunsaturates have earned their good reputation because they lower blood cholesterol levels.

A fourth kind of fat we get from foods is *monounsaturated fat,* which is found in greatest amounts in olive oil and peanut oil. For many years, researchers thought monounsaturated fat was neutral—neither raising nor lowering blood

Know how to tell the good and the bad from the ugly.

Snack crackers made with palm or coconut oil have twice the saturated fat of beef.

Unsaturated fats can lower your cholesterol.

Monounsaturated fats lower only the bad kind of cholesterol.

cholesterol levels. But recent research performed by Scott M. Grundy, M.D., Ph.D., director of the Center for Human Nutrition at the University of Texas Southwestern Medical Center at Dallas, has revealed that it does, in fact, lower blood cholesterol.

Not only that, but monounsaturated fat manages to lower LDL blood cholesterol while it leaves HDL blood cholesterol alone. But polyunsaturated fat reduces both. Why does this matter? As you may remember from earlier chapters, LDL cholesterol in the blood causes the most harm to the arteries, so you want to get rid of as much of that as you can. But HDL cholesterol appears to act like a scavenger, removing harmful cholesterol from the blood, so you want to hang onto it.

Monounsaturated fat has also been linked to lower blood pressure, even among obese men who might otherwise be at risk, according to a recent study performed by the Stanford Center for Research in Disease Prevention at the Stanford University School of Medicine.

The *omega-3 fatty acids* we talked about earlier are another kind of "good" fat. Found mostly in fish and shellfish, they are a special class of polyunsaturates that have also been shown to reduce blood cholesterol levels.

So there you have it—the different kinds of fat most relevant to your quest toward lower-fat eating. Now how do you know when to reach for what?

A fat-reduction plan.

For starters, the first rule is to reduce the total amount of fat in your diet to 30 percent of your daily calories, a figure recommended by the AHA and many major dietary fat experts. That means if you eat about 2,000 calories a day, only about 600 of them should be derived from fat—any kind of fat. Of that 30 percent, you should strive to get only about 10 percent from saturated fat. The remaining 20 percent should be divided among polyunsaturates and monounsaturates.

The food eaten in a typical day by most Amer-

Where's the Cholesterol?

Dietary cholesterol, especially when combined with saturated fat, can raise blood cholesterol levels. The American Heart Association recommends that Americans eat no more than 300 milligrams of dietary cholesterol per day. How much cholesterol is in your particular passion?

Food	Portion	Cholesterol (mg)
Beef liver, fried	3 oz.	410
Beef liver, braised	3 oz.	331
Eggs, whole	1 medium	274
Shrimp	8 large	86
Lobster	1 cup	104
	3 oz.	61
Turkey, dark meat, roasters, no skin	3 oz.	95
Pork, fresh, leg, whole, lean, roasted	3 oz.	80
Chicken, dark meat, broilers or fryers, roasted, no skin	3 oz.	79
Beef, lean, ground, broiled medium	3 oz.	74
Fish, fatty (sockeye salmon)	3 oz.	74
Turkey, light meat, roasters, no skin	3 oz.	73
Chicken, light meat, fryers, no skin	3 oz.	72
Fish, lean (haddock), cooked, dry heat	3 oz.	63
Ham, cured, extra lean, roasted	3 oz.	48
Frankfurters, all beef, 30% fat, 8 per pound	1	35
Tuna, white, packed in water, drained	3 oz.	35
Milk, whole	1 cup	33
Cheese, cottage, 4% fat	1 cup	31
Cheese, cheddar	1 oz.	30
Ice cream	½ cup	30
Butter	1 tbsp.	20
Cheese, "light," 1% fat	1 oz.	20
Bacon, cooked crisp	3 slices	16
Cheese, mozzarella, part-skim	1 oz.	16
Cheese, cottage, 1% fat	1 cup	10
Milk, skim	1 cup	4
Peanut butter	2 tbsp.	0

SOURCE: Adapted from USDA Agriculture Handbooks nos. 8–1, 8–4, 8–5, 8–10, 8–13, 8–15 and 8–16 (Washington, D.C.: U.S. Department of Agriculture).

icans now contains about 40 percent fat, with a heavy emphasis on saturated fat. So what health experts are encouraging us to do is reduce all the fat we eat. And when you must eat fat, try to replace saturated fat with a more benign form like polyunsaturated or monounsaturated. You might want to switch from butter, a saturated fat, to soft margarine, a mostly polyunsaturated fat.

Keep your cholesterol under 300 mg per day.

As far as dietary cholesterol is concerned, the AHA advises that you eat no more than 300 milligrams per day. (See the table, "Where's the Cholesterol?" on page 71 for the major sources of dietary cholesterol.) One of the best ways to do this is to avoid eating the foods highest in cholesterol, like eggs and liver.

But certain kinds of high-cholesterol shellfish, such as shrimp, may occasionally be okay, because they contain omega-3 fatty acids, according to Dr. William Connor, the Oregon Health Sciences University researcher who has done some of the most important work on fish and blood cholesterol. That doesn't mean you should eat a lot of high-cholesterol shellfish—it just means that in moderation it may not be as harmful to eat as medical experts once thought.

How to Figure Out the Fat in Your Diet

The next logical question you may be asking yourself is how in the world you can figure out milligrams of cholesterol and percentages of fat in the many foods you eat. To help you, we've included tables with this chapter that give you the percentages of calories from fat and milligrams of cholesterol in many common foods.

Choose fats and oils carefully.

There is also a list of all the different kinds of fats and oils you might use in cooking or see on prepared food labels. It lets you know which are rich in saturated fat and which contain more polyunsaturated or monounsaturated fat.

But since every table has limits, you may be wondering how you can figure out the percentage

Fats and Oils: Which Should You Reach for First?

Adding some fat to a recipe? Choosing a salad oil? Looking for a spread for your bread? You should use all fats and oils sparingly, advise dietary fat experts, but if you do reach for one, grab from among the ones that are least saturated. Here's how they measure up—from least saturated to most, best choice to worst.

Rapeseed oil (canola oil)

Safflower oil

Sunflower oil

Corn oil

Olive oil

Hydrogenated sunflower oil

Margarine, liquid, bottled

Margarine, soft, tub

Sesame oil

Soybean oil

Margarine, stick

Peanut oil

Cottonseed oil

Lard

Beef tallow

Palm oil

Butter

Cocoa butter

Palm kernel oil

Coconut oil

of calories from fat in foods not listed on our table. It's really very simple, as long as the food label lists the calories and grams of fat per serving. (Most do, and many more are starting to, as people get more concerned about the nutritional content of their foods.)

It's just basic mathematics. A gram of fat con-

How to Figure the Percentage of Calories from Fat

You're standing in the supermarket aisle, trying to figure out how much fat is in the product you're holding. It lists grams of fat—but that doesn't help. What you need to know is the percentage of calories from fat in the product so you can see how it lines up with the American Heart Association's recommendation to get only 30 percent of your calories from fat. This chart gives you an easy way to do that. Bring along your pocket calculator for quick estimating.

Whole Milk—A Sample Label
Nutrition Information per Serving

Serving size	1 cup
Servings per container	4
Calories	150
Protein	8 grams
Carbohydrates	11 grams
Fat	8 grams

1. Multiply the number of grams of fat (8) by the number of calories in a gram of fat (9) to get the number of fat calories: $8 \times 9 = 72$.

2. Divide the number of fat calories (72) by the number of total calories (150) to get the percentage of calories from fat: $72 \div 150 = 48\%$.

Multiply times 9.

tains 9 calories. If a serving of the food you want to eat contains 5 grams of fat, you multiply 9 times 5. Now you know the number of fat calories is 45. If a serving contains 90 calories in total, you can figure out that almost 50 percent of its calories are derived from fat.

The U.S. Food and Drug Administration is working on a regulation that would require manufacturers who list the cholesterol content of their products to also list the amount of saturated and polyunsaturated fat they contain. If approved, that

How Fat Is Your Food?

The American Heart Association recommends that you cut back the fat in your diet from the typical 40 percent of calories to 30 percent. But how do you know the percentage of fat in an average meal? This chart will help you figure it out. Try to choose foods that are close to 30 percent fat or less. Or, if you do choose foods higher in fat like many cheeses and meats, eat them in smaller portions and combine them with low-fat foods. Add a small amount of meat to a casserole that includes low-fat rice, noodles, vegetables or beans, for example. All meats here are trimmed of fat, unless otherwise noted.

Food	Percentage of Calories from Fat
Beef	
Hot dog, all beef, about 30% fat by weight	81
T-bone, choice, broiled, untrimmed	68
Ground beef, regular, broiled medium	65
Porterhouse, choice, broiled, untrimmed	64
Ground beef, lean, broiled medium	61
Ground beef, extra lean, select, broiled medium	58
Round steak, select, broiled, untrimmed	58
Flank steak, choice, braised	51
Rib, whole, select, roasted	49
Porterhouse, choice, broiled	45
T-bone, choice, broiled	44
Bottom round, choice, braised	40
Sirloin, wedge-bone, choice, broiled	39
Tenderloin, select, broiled	38
Bottom round, select, braised	37
Chuck arm pot roast, select, braised	36
Top loin, select, broiled	36
Sirloin, wedge-bone, select, broiled	35
Tip round, select, roasted	33
Eye of round, select, roasted	30
Top round steak, select, broiled	27
Lamb	
Rib roast, roasted	55
Blade chop, broiled	50
Arm chop, braised	47
Loin chop, broiled	42
Sirloin half of leg, roasted	42
Shank half of leg, roasted	34
Foreshank, braised	30
Pork	
Bacon, 3 medium slices	78
Spareribs, braised	69
Loin, center rib, untrimmed, braised	67
Loin, blade, roasted	62
Loin, whole, roasted	52

(continued)

How Fat Is Your Food?—Continued

Food	Percentage of Calories from Fat
Pork—Continued	
Loin, top loin, roasted	51
Ham leg, rump half, roasted	44
Ham leg, shank half, roasted	44
Loin, tenderloin, roasted	26
Poultry	
Duck, domesticated, meat only, roasted	50
Chicken, broiler or fryer, dark meat only, roasted	43
Chicken, broiler or fryer, breast meat only, roasted	19
Turkey, breast meat only, roasted	5
Veal	
Rib roast, roasted	40
Loin chop, braised	38
Blade steak, braised	31
Sirloin chop, braised	30
Arm steak, braised	25
Veal cutlet, fried	23
Seafood	
Salmon, sockeye, cooked, dry heat	46
Flounder or sole, cooked, dry heat	12
Shrimp, cooked, moist heat	10
Tuna, light, packed in water	3
Dairy	
Half-and-half, 1 tbsp.	76
Cheese, Swiss, 1 oz.	64
Egg, 1	64
Mozzarella, part-skim, 1 oz.	55
Milk, whole, 1 cup	48
Ice cream, vanilla, regular (10% fat), 1 cup	47
Cheese, cottage, creamed, 1 cup	38
Milk, low-fat (2%), 1 cup	34
Yogurt, low-fat, plain, 8 oz.	21
Cheese, cottage, low-fat (1%), 1 cup	12
Sherbet, orange, 1 cup	12
Milk, skim 1 cup	4
Fruits and Vegetables	
Avocado, ½ fruit	80
Coconut meat, raw, shredded, ½ cup	79
Apple, 1	5
Banana, 1	4
Carrot, 1	4
Beans, snap green, cooked, ½ cup	3
Orange, 1	2
Potato, baked, 1	1

Food	Percentage of Calories from Fat
Grains and Beans	
Bread, whole wheat, 1 slice	12
Rice, brown, 1 cup	4
Spaghetti, 1 cup	4
Kidney beans, 1 cup	3
Lentils, 1 cup	3
Split peas, 1 cup	3
Nuts	
Peanuts, dried, 1 oz.	73
Peanut butter, smooth, 1 tbsp.	72
Snacks	
Potato chips, 10	60
Chocolate bar, milk, plain, 1 oz.	52
Doughnut, cake-type, 1	48
Popcorn, plain, air-popped, 1 cup	0

ADAPTED FROM: USDA Handbooks nos. 8–1, 8–5, 8–9, 8–10, 8–12, 8–13 and 8–15, and Home and Gardens Bulletin No. 72 (Washington, D.C.: U.S. Department of Agriculture).

Journal of Food Science, vol. 51, 1986.

Journal of Food Science, vol. 49, 1986.

NOTE: All meats are 3 ounces, trimmed, unless otherwise noted.

should also make it easier for you to sort out what kind of fat you're eating, as well as how much of it is in a product.

Launch a Fat Attack

Although learning how much and what kinds of fat are in foods is an important first step on the road to lower-fat eating, it's only the beginning. Your real efforts will begin when you start adapting the foods you presently eat to suit your new eating style. The best place to start is with foods that are obvious sources of fat—meat, cheese, eggs, milk and spreads like butter, mayonnaise and peanut butter. Alas, some of our favorite foods!

But don't worry—we're not asking you to give them all up, only to redefine your relationship

Learn how to have your cake and eat it, too.

with them. This is an area where many of you have probably already made strides. Who hasn't, cut back a bit on red meat—known to be high in saturated fat—or tried switching from butter to margarine at least part of the time? Here are some other creative strategies.

Meat. There are several ways to go when you're trying to reduce the amount of saturated fat you get from meat. For many, the easiest way to start is by trimming all visible fat from meats and choosing leaner cuts of red meat. (See the table, "How Fat Is Your Food?" on page 75 for the percentage of calories from fat in various cuts of beef, pork, lamb and veal.)

Trim the fat.

A simple example is to eat more flank steak, also known as London broil, instead of fattier steaks. Choose the leanest ground beef you can find, or better still, opt for ground round or ground sirloin, which are much lower in fat than other kinds of ground beef. And start trying beef graded "Select" instead of "Choice" or "Prime." It tends to be much lower in fat than the others.

Swap T-bone for London broil.

Another easy way to cut fat is simply to eat smaller portions of meat. That may sound depressing if you picture a tiny, lonely cube of meat on your plate—so don't. Instead, imagine meat sliced, chopped and slivered into casseroles and stews so it becomes one more ingredient instead of the star attraction on your plate. There are several cookbooks available now that feature low-fat recipes using meat this way. (See the box, "Stroke-Buster Cookbooks," on page 96 for some recommendations.)

Chop, sliver and slice.

A third way to reduce the fat you get from meat is to eat it at fewer meals a day. As a general rule, try to work toward eating only 6 ounces or less of meat per day, a guideline recommended by the AHA. The Connors suggest that you start by cutting meat from your breakfast menu, then slowly from your lunch, too. If you find yourself stuck at the deli counter yearning for a corned beef or salami sandwich, choose turkey- or chicken-based luncheon meat instead.

Leaning more toward poultry and fish, which have less fat than red meat, is a fourth way to manipulate your eating style to reduce fat. Just remember that it's better to use chicken in casseroles and stews than to roast or bake it with the skin on—since the skin does contain the lion's share of fat. (See, there is a way around dry, skinless chicken!)

Lean toward fish and away from meat.

Finally, consider having a few meatless dinners per week. In place of meat, substitute other protein foods such as beans, grains and other high-fiber, filling foods. A good example of this is a meatless chili, using kidney beans, corn and rice. The cookbooks we recommend contain many recipes that help you do this creatively.

Cheese. This is a food with a lot of misconceptions surrounding it. Many people plan meatless meals and substitute cheese-based dishes, thinking they're better off because they're avoiding red meat. In fact, cheese is a worse choice in terms of saturated fat and cholesterol. Most regular cheeses get about 70 percent of their calories from fat! The other problem with cheese is our tendency to eat it as a snack food. It's so easy for the ounces to pile up without our being conscious of it.

But despite the bad news, there's also some good news in the cheese world today—the introduction of new lower-fat hard cheeses and sliced sandwich cheeses. These cheeses taste so good you don't feel deprived, and they're a good way to start reducing your fat intake. Look in your regular cheese department at the supermarket, or try specialty food stores or cheese shops, which may carry a larger variety of low-fat brands. Since some of the lower-fat cheeses are made from vegetable oils rather than butterfat, you'll be happy to know that you may be reducing your saturated fat intake and substituting polyunsaturated fat in the process.

Go for the new low-fat cheeses.

Mix high-fat and low-fat cheeses for super taste.

The Family Heart Study made a particular effort to address the problems of eating too much cheese because the researchers found that so many participants loved it. Among their suggestions to families: Mix a lower-fat cheese like part-skim or imitation mozzarella with higher-fat cheeses like cheddar, to get the flavor without all the saturated fat and cholesterol. And use Parmesan cheese for flavoring. Even though it's high in fat, we tend to use it in smaller quantities.

Look for cheeses that contain 6 g or less of fat per ounce.

Read labels, and look for cheeses that generally contain 6 g or less of fat per ounce. You can go a little higher than that (up to 9 g per ounce) if the cheese is made from skim milk and vegetable oil, since the fat would be the polyunsaturated kind instead of saturated. Eventually, when you feel comfortable with lower-fat cheeses, you may want to try truly low-fat cheeses, which contain 3 g of fat or less per ounce—that's the recommendation of the AHA.

Eggs. Although eggs are a good source of protein and other nutrients, they're also one of the most potent sources of dietary cholesterol around. One egg at breakfast delivers 270 mg of dietary cholesterol—almost the entire 300-mg limit recommended by experts for the entire day. And that does not even take into account the additional dietary cholesterol that we get from meat, cheese, butter and other dairy products. Or the egg that is mixed into prepared foods like baked goods and egg noodles.

There are basically two simple ways to confront the egg dilemma. First, try to limit yourself to two whole eggs per week (maybe as a treat on a Saturday or Sunday morning). And for recipes that call for eggs, substitute two egg whites for each whole egg specified. Since the cholesterol in eggs is centered in the yolk, the whites don't present a problem. And you'll be amazed at how little you'll notice the difference between recipes with and without yolks.

You can fool even the most dedicated egg lovers this way. But if you do run into some balking, try going half-and-half. If the recipe calls for two eggs, for example, use one whole and two egg whites. You can do this when preparing omelet and scrambled eggs, too. Remember, slow, gradual change is the best route to permanent change.

Substitute two egg whites for each whole egg in a recipe.

Milk and cream. We've talked a little about how to cut back on the fat in milk by starting with a change to 2 percent milk, and then gradually moving on to 1 percent and skim. This is especially easy to do in recipes, so even if your family rebels against the change in drinking milk, they may not even notice the change in cooking.

Switch to 2 percent milk to get started.

There's been some confusion in recent years over the percentages cited when you're talking about various milks. That's because milk makers list the percentage of fat by weight on their labels to distinguish between their products. But what you need to know is the percentage of calories from fat in the various milks. Whole milk, for example, which is a little over 3 percent fat by weight, derives almost 50 percent of its calories from fat! Milk that's 2 percent fat by weight gets about 34 percent of its calories from fat. (See the table, "How Fat Is Your Food?" on page 75 for the percentage of fat calories in other dairy products.)

In the coffee creamer department, beware of nondairy products. Most of them are made with palm or coconut oils, the two vegetable oils high in saturated fat. Better to use a low-fat milk or nonfat dried milk.

Avoid nondairy coffee creamers.

If you're a fan of half-and-half or cream in your coffee, see if you can slowly wean yourself toward whole milk. Half-and-half and cream are almost completely fat. Once you've grown accustomed to whole milk, you may be able to make further strides toward 2 percent or even lower-fat milk.

One low-fat dairy product that's easy to live with is yogurt. It can be a nice alternative to higher-fat sour cream in recipes and dips as long as it's the low-fat or skim variety. The cookbooks we recommend use yogurt in creative ways as a substitute. You might also try frozen low-fat yogurt as a substitute for ice cream.

Speaking of ice cream, we wish we could duck this one—but we can't. Even regular ice cream gets about 50 percent of its calories from fat. The gourmet ice creams are even worse. If you're really addicted, cut back slowly. Fortunately, there are truly a lot of good-tasting, low-fat, frozen dessert alternatives to ice cream. Sherbet is much lower in fat, not to mention the nonfat sorbets and frozen fruit bars flooding the market.

Spreads. Butter . . . mayonnaise . . . peanut butter. For many people, they're the only reason to eat bread. But we hardly need to tell you that these spreads are the purest kind of fat around. Alas, they're also the foods some people hold dearest to their hearts. So go slowly in this area, because rebellion can result (your own or your family's) if you move too quickly.

Nutritionists in the Family Heart Study suggest that if the taste of margarine is too big a change to tolerate all at once, then begin by using mostly margarine—with a little bit of butter for flavoring—in recipes. Don't try to switch the butter on the table right away if you really can't bear the thought. But gradually try to make an almost complete change from butter to margarine.

What kind of margarines are best? Choose the soft-tub margarines, since these are the kinds highest in polyunsaturated fat. Look for a liquid oil, such as corn, safflower or sunflower, as the first ingredient on your margarine label. The nutrition information should indicate that there's at least twice as much polyunsaturated fat as saturated fat in it.

But whether you're spreading margarine or butter, learn the fine art of "scraping" it onto your breads and muffins, advise the nutritionists in the Family Heart Study. Or better still, use a little jam or jelly instead of fatty spread. Although jams con-

The ice cream alternative.

Soft-tub margarines are the best kind of spreads.

Substitute jams and jellies for butter.

tain sugar, they have fewer calories and no fat.

In the mayonnaise area, most of us have been rescued from despair with the introduction of imitation mayonnaises. Although marketed for their low-calorie appeal, they also have a much lower fat content.

Peanut butter, like cheese, is also high on Americans' lists as an all-time favorite snack—on crackers or right out of the jar. Although high in fat, it's much less saturated than animal fat, so it's still a better choice for a sandwich than most cheese and meat. Nevertheless, it's very high in total fat (about 75 percent of its calories come from fat), so the main change you want to make here is to use it in meals instead of as a frequent snack.

Oils. Most oils, like safflower, rapeseed (sold as Puritan Oil in your supermarket), sunflower, soybean, cottonseed and corn, are high in polyunsaturated fat and are definitely a better choice than butter for cooking. But use them sparingly, since they are still fats.

Olive oil and peanut oil are both high in monounsaturated fats, so go ahead and use them if you prefer their flavor.

Olive and peanut oils are better choices than others.

Coconut and palm oil, the two vegetable oils tremendously high in saturated fat, should be off your list completely. Both are being used extensively right now by many food manufacturers because they're among the cheapest oils available on the market. Sometimes they're hard to notice, because they're listed in parentheses after the general term "vegetable oils." Our eyes tend to pass quickly over this because we assume all vegetable oils are high in polyunsaturated fat.

Be on the lookout for coconut and palm oil in such products as cereals, breads, shortenings, whipped toppings, nondairy coffee creamers, cake frostings, bread stuffings, frozen dinner entreés, various cookies, crackers and chips. Of course, not all food manufacturers use these ingredients, so

Avoid coconut and palm oils.

check and choose products that list acceptable oils.

Better still, try to substitute products that don't use fat at all, or use it only in very tiny amounts. There are many kinds of low-fat crackers and other munchies such as matzoh, crispbreads, popcorn, pretzels and soda crackers.

Shake the Salt Habit

Most of the salt that we eat comes from two sources: the stuff we add to our food willingly and the stuff manufacturers put into their products whether we like it or not. In both cases, it adds up to a lot of sodium—frequently between 4,000 and 5,000 mg a day. Experts tell us we should be cutting back to between 1,000 and 3,000 mg per day. But how?

Fortunately, our whole country has become salt-wise over the last decade, since health professionals started spreading the word about salt being closely allied to high blood pressure. There are now a variety of foods on the market that emphasize lower salt content. You probably already use many of them.

Leave the salt shaker in the cupboard.

If you haven't made any effort to cut down your salt consumption, however, it's important to move slowly in this area. Your taste buds will get used to eating less salt (and in fact, will come to prefer it, according to studies), but give it time. Begin by trying not to add salt to foods at the table. Taste foods before you salt them. You may find that you don't need any extra salt.

Your next plan of attack should focus on cooking. Try to cut back on the amount of salt you've traditionally used in recipes—you'll be surprised to notice that, in some instances, less doesn't seem to make a difference. When cooking pasta, rice, noodles and hot cereals, for example, you may discover that they taste exactly the same with or without added salt.

Experiment with herbs.

You should also experiment with herb and spice salt substitutes in recipes and on the table. These mixtures fool your palate by incorporating ingredients like citrus flavors, which manage to excite the taste buds that usually respond to salt, says Judith Benn Hurley, a cookbook author who specializes in healthy foods. "The herbs in these mixtures also play a role in helping you not to miss salt. They bloom in your mouth and keep different taste buds busy." (See the table, "Spice Up Your Life," on page 85 for some suggestions for salt substitutes.)

But be sure to consult your doctor before using potassium chloride, another popular salt substitute. Although potassium has been noted to have a favorable effect on blood pressure, your doctor should know before you add it to your diet this way, since too much potassium can be dangerous. That's especially true if you're being treated

Spice Up Your Life

Looking for an herb and spice salt substitute as a way to cut back on salt? Mix up your own or check out one of the five herb and spice substitutes evaluated below by the Rodale Food Center. If you're interested in trying potassium chloride as a salt substitute, be sure to check with your doctor first. Too much potassium chloride can be dangerous, especially if you're being treated for such conditions as diabetes, heart disease or kidney disease.

Product	Taste	Aroma	Appearance	Comments
American Heart Association Herb Seasonings	Good, spicy, zesty flavors	Good and full	Nice shapes in lemon herb flavor	Original, salad and lemon herb flavors
Deep Roots	Good, herbal flavor; Mexican very hot	Herbal	Wholesome, green	Mexican, whole herb, Italian flavors
Instead of salt	Good, well-chosen flavors; should be added before cooking	Good and full, especially vegetable flavor	Nice colors	All-Purpose, Fish, Chicken, Beef and Vegetable flavors
Mrs. Dash	Excellent, well-balanced, peppery citrus flavor	Peppery and robust	Colorful	Good, low-cal topping for baked potatoes; low-pepper and no-garlic flavors
Vegit	Good, slightly yeasty	Herbal and yeasty	Powdery	Good on popcorn

for such conditions as diabetes, heart disease or kidney disease.

As you begin to use less salt at the table and in cooking, you'll probably start to notice where the rest of the excess salt in your diet comes from. And it's usually processed foods. Suddenly those bouillon cubes or the canned soup you mix into a recipe tastes too salty. But when you're in doubt about how much salt is in a product, turn to the label. The higher it appears on the ingredient list, the more salt is in the product. And if a label lists nutrient information, look at the sodium content. Fortunately, many food manufacturers are making lower-sodium versions of their products. So start experimenting with them now.

Check the salt content of processed foods.

You should also try to lean more toward fresh foods, which usually contain very little salt, and watch out for condiments, which are notoriously high in salt. These include ketchup, steak sauce, barbecue sauce, soy sauce, Worcestershire sauce, pickles, pickle relish and mustard. Substitute chopped onions, green peppers, lemon juice and other flavorings.

Changing Your Relationship to Sugar

Sugar isn't nearly the cardiovascular health problem that fat is—but it still needs your attention, particularly if you're overweight. Cutting down on sugar can take hundreds of empty calories out of your diet, and it's not that hard to do. There are three specific routes to follow.

Three ways to cut back on sugar.

First, you might try eating fruits instead of sweets when a craving for sugar strikes your taste buds. It may not work every time, but even part of the time is a step ahead. You might also begin adding less sugar to foods at the table, especially in hot and cold drinks or on top of cereal or fruit. And try substituting unsweetened drinks, like seltzer and club soda with a twist of lemon or lime, for sodas and other highly sugared drinks. Go as slowly as you need to—remember, the idea is to keep your taste buds from rebelling.

Second, reduce the amount of sugar you use in recipes by at least one-third. As with salt, you'll be surprised at how little difference it makes to add less sugar than the recipe specifies.

Cut the sugar in your recipes by one-third.

Third, try to avoid foods that add a lot of hidden sugar, like salad dressing, soup, spaghetti sauce and condiments such as ketchup and relish. Or just use less of them. And when you're reading labels looking for hidden sugar, keep in mind that sugar is a product with many names. Among them: sucrose, glucose, dextrose, fructose, maltose, lactose, honey, corn syrup, high-fructose corn syrup, molasses and maple sugar. If any of those terms appear among the first three ingredients on a product's label, it's probably high in sugar.

A word on artificial sweeteners: Even though many people swear by them as a way to avoid sugar and lose weight, a study of 78,000 women showed that the artificial sweetener users fared no better than the real sugar users in terms of the amount of weight lost. In fact, more artificial sweetener users *gained* weight than nonusers. That's not to say these sweeteners don't have a place in your new, lower-sugar diet—just keep in mind that they may not be enough to help you lose weight.

Artificial sweeteners can't do it alone.

Bring on the Fish

When you combine fish's low-fat reputation with the discovery that it also contains omega-3 fatty acids, you come up with an ideal protein food to replace fattier meats on the dinner table.

Fish: the ideal protein food.

Which fish should you reach for fastest? Herring, mackerel, salmon, bluefish, tuna, whitefish, sturgeon, lake trout, sardines and anchovies are among the best finfish sources of omega-3s. But bass, carp, halibut, hake, pollack, eel, pompano, rockfish, shark, rainbow trout, cod, flounder, perch, haddock, sole and swordfish are also good. And shellfish like crab, shrimp, oysters, clams, scallops and lobster also contain omega-3s. That's good news for people who may be avoiding shellfish because some kinds—shrimp, for example—are high in cholesterol. The omega-3s in shellfish seem to negate cholesterol's ill effects on the arteries, say the experts.

How much fish should you eat? Studies show that as little as two fish meals a week can exert a positive effect on your cardiovascular system. So become a regular at the fish store or fish counter at your supermarket.

Two fish dishes a week can enhance your cardiovascular system.

Many people shy away from fish because they don't know how to prepare it without adding a lot of calories and fat from breading and frying, or cooking in butter. But fish is an ideal food to poach, broil or bake. You can use water, juices or perhaps a little wine to retain moistness and, for additional flavoring, don't forget to add your favorite herbs and spices.

If you have a microwave oven, you should know that fish is one of the things it does best. The key to doing it well, says cookbook author Judith Benn Hurley, is to be sure it's at room temperature before starting. "If fish is chilled, it creates a texture problem," she says. "Because it takes so long for the microwaves to warm the outside, you wind up overcooking." Hurley suggests trying this quick and easy recipe: Smother the fish in chopped tomatoes and basil and microwave on full power for about 4 minutes.

Try beans, soybeans and walnuts if you hate fish.

A word for those of you who positively, absolutely can't stand fish. There are some nonfish sources of omega-3 fatty acids, including dry beans, soybeans and walnuts. Wheat germ, soybean and walnut oils also contain omega-3s. Spinach, broccoli and cauliflower contain traces. Some more exotic sources coming onto the market are a Mediterranean vegetable called purslane, and canola or rapeseed oil. As for omega-3 fish-oil supplements, health professionals are divided on whether people should be taking them. But one thing is clear: They shouldn't serve as a substitute for a healthy diet.

Feast on Fiber

As you begin cutting back on the amount of high-fat foods you eat, you'll eventually need to supplement your meals with other foods. The ideal foods to add are legumes (beans and lentils), various grain-based foods like pasta, rice, bread and noodles, and more vegetables and fruits. All are excellent sources of fiber and complex carbohydrates. And legumes and grains are good sources of lean protein, too.

High-fiber, high-carbohydrate foods fill you up with fewer calories and much less fat, and they may help control your blood cholesterol and blood sugar levels. But because, for most of us, they've played only supporting roles in our present way of eating, it's a challenge to add them in greater quantities to our menus.

Make legumes and grains major players on your family's menus.

It all goes back to that idea of taste preferences. As kids, we may not have eaten these foods very much, so we haven't formed habits and eating rituals around them.

Think of how many different ways you know to prepare ground beef. But with the exception of a single dish—chili, for example—do you hold dear to your heart any other recipe that includes kidney beans? Most of us would probably say no. And how many of us have virtually wiped breads, noodles and other starchy foods off our menus, fearing that they would make us fat? Sabine Artaud-Wild, a registered dietitian who worked on the Family Heart Study nutrition staff, says convincing the people who participated in the study that high-fiber, complex-carbohydrate foods like bread and noodles were not the "bad guys" was one of the most difficult jobs they had.

Breads and noodles do not make you fat.

Even when you overcome the familiarity

problem and realize that high-fiber, high-carbohydrate foods are not fattening (as long as you don't cover them with fatty spreads and sauces!), there are other obstacles, says the University of Oregon's Sonja Connor. High-fiber, high-carbohydrate foods are just beginning to be transformed into convenience foods. You can't always find ready-made, healthfully prepared, high-carbohydrate foods in your local deli case. "Yet, it would be so easy to do," says Connor. How? Ready-made pasta and macaroni salads, for example, can be made with low-fat, low-cholesterol dressings instead of the creamy, egg-laden mixtures most deli counters use now.

A new generation of cookbooks is making stroke-busting diets a reality.

The other difficulty in adding fiber, says Connor, is the lack of a wide variety of recipes using beans, grains and vegetables in tasty, delicious ways that are designed for the American palate. Fortunately, a new generation of cookbooks is solving the problem. (See the box, "Stroke-Buster Cookbooks," on page 96.) Try one new recipe a week, suggests Connor, and you'll soon have a symphonic repertoire. But remember to move slowly. Overwhelm yourself or your family with too many seemingly strange new food tastes and textures and you're asking for all-out rebellion— or at least a speedy retreat to your local fast food eatery.

Learn from other cultures.

Fortunately, many other cultures have used high-fiber foods as staples in their diet for centuries. Even more fortunately, some of these cuisines—Mexican, Oriental and Italian, for example—are America's favorites. So one thing you can do even before you try new recipes is to simply remove some of the fat we as a culture have added to many ethnic dishes. Spaghetti sauce and chili, for example, can be prepared using much less meat, without losing the flavor we enjoy. Or try making a meatless chili or spaghetti sauce occasionally and concentrate on herbs, spices and vegetables for flavoring.

And for those of you who are resistant to the idea of adding more beans to your recipes because they tend to cause excess gas, try degassing dried beans this way: Soak them for about 3 hours, boil for about 30 minutes (add fresh water if needed) and discard the water. For those of you on very busy schedules, use canned beans, which are fully cooked, very convenient and, again, lacking in propulsive properties.

Make your beans socially acceptable.

But cooking high-fiber, high-carbohydrate foods while cutting back on the quantities of meat and cheese you eat will probably mean that you prepare many more stews, soups and low-fat sauces. You add small amounts of meat for flavoring, while increasing the amounts of vegetables, beans and starchy foods. Once again, a microwave oven is a handy way to prepare food this way, says Hurley. To make a stew, for example, put together ingredients the night before and cook them quickly in your microwave. Then leave them in your refrigerator until dinnertime the next day. By that time, all the flavors will have had time to blend and you can simply heat it up after a busy day.

Cooking vegetables well in the microwave is simply a matter of making sure pieces are nearly the same size, says Hurley. For vegetables like broccoli and asparagus, which have tough, thick stalks, arrange the stalks in a circle, with the delicate buds facing toward the middle. This will ensure that the stalks get a more intense cooking. For potatoes, cook quickly in the microwave, then broil them in your oven for a few minutes to crisp the skins.

Zap your veggies.

How much fiber should you add to your diet? The U.S. Department of Agriculture recommends around 30 grams a day, eaten in a wide variety of high-fiber foods, including whole grain breads, cereals and pastas; vegetables and fruits; and beans and legumes. (See the table, "Feast on Fiber," on page 92 to see which foods contain the most.)

Boost your fiber to 30 grams a day.

Feast on Fiber

How much fiber should you eat? Most Americans eat only 12 to 15 grams per day, although experts say we should be eating 25 to 35 grams. Here are some of the richest sources. When looking for the fiber content on product labels, make sure the listing is for *dietary* fiber. Crude fiber, an older measurement, is still sometimes used, but is less accurate.

Food	Portion	Total Dietary Fiber (g)
Grain and Grain Products		
Bran, oat	⅓ cup	7.8
Bran Flakes, ready-to-eat*	⅔ cup	4.6
Bran, corn	1 tbsp.	3.0
Bread, pita, whole wheat	1	2.6
Oatmeal, dry	⅓ cup	2.4
Bread, whole wheat	1 slice	2.0
Bran, wheat, crude	1 tbsp.	1.5
Fruits		
Figs, dried	3	9.5
Blackberries	½ cup	4.5
Pear	1 medium	4.3
Dates, dried	5	3.6
Orange	1 medium	3.1

When you're looking for fiber content on package labels, however, make sure the listing is for *dietary* fiber, not crude fiber. Crude fiber is an older and less accurate measurement.

Lose Weight Naturally

As you shift from an eating style that is high in fat, sugar and salt toward one that's high in complex carbohydrates, fiber and lean protein, you'll probably find that weight comes off without the help of a special weight-reducing diet. That's because your new way of eating is naturally lower in calories than the old way. Besides, most special diets don't work anyway, simply because people go "on" a diet but don't really make a lifetime commitment

Food	Portion	Total Dietary Fiber (g)
Apple, with skin	1 medium	2.8
Strawberries	1 cup	2.8
Banana	1 medium	1.8
Melons, cantaloupe, cubed	1 cup	1.3
Raisins	¼ cup	1.1
Legumes and Nuts		
Beans, kidney, cooked	½ cup	9.0
Beans, pinto, cooked	½ cup	8.9
Lima beans, cooked, drained	½ cup	6.6
Chick-peas, canned, drained	½ cup	6.5
Peanuts, roasted	1 oz.	2.6
Peanut butter, chunky	1 tbsp.	1.1
Vegetables		
Potato, raw, flesh and skin	1 medium	3.0
Carrot, raw	1 medium	2.3
Broccoli, raw, chopped	½ cup	1.2
Cabbage, red, raw	½ cup	0.7

SOURCE: Adapted from provisional data supplied by USDA Nutrient Data, Beltsville, Md.
*Values may vary among different brands of this type of cereal.

to changing their eating habits. So, when they've lost weight and then go "off" the diet, they gradually go back to eating the way they did before—and the pounds pile on again. If you're slowly making permanent changes in the way you eat, this shouldn't happen to you.

But, depending on how overweight you are or how firmly ingrained your eating habits are, you may want and need some extra help in learning to change what the experts call your *eating behavior.* That means becoming aware of how, why and when you eat—or overeat—and learning to control or change that behavior. Here's a selection of tips from weight-loss experts across the country. But don't feel you have to follow *all* these ideas to lose weight. Just pick and choose from among the strategies to find the ones that work best for you.

Learn how, why and when you eat.

Keep a food diary. This handy record-keeping device is simply a log of what you eat, along with the time and place that eating occurred. Some people also record what they were doing while eating (reading, talking, watching TV) and how they were feeling.

Weight-loss experts say this is one of the most useful tools you can use to come to grips with your eating behavior. That's because most of us tend to underestimate how much we're eating. And a diary helps you get a more accurate picture. A diary also makes you aware of the quality of foods you're eating so you can keep an eye on your fat and sugar intake.

A diary keeps you honest.

But perhaps most important, a food diary reveals your eating patterns—not just preferences for certain foods, but times of the day or days of the week (such as weekends) when you overeat. Or people you tend to overeat with. Or places (like in front of the TV) where most of your overeating occurs. Finding out when you're most vulnerable is the first step in exerting some control over those times.

Learn your food cues. Through a diary, you can learn food "cues"—those things, places or times that seem to instigate eating. And one of the biggest is probably your refrigerator. How many times do you walk by and just open the door with no particular purpose in mind? Yet once you look inside, you probably find something to eat.

Making the unconscious conscious will put you in control.

Watching television seems to be another potent food cue for many people, as is preparing meals. Others get the urge while they're on the telephone. Your food diary should help reveal these cues. And once you're conscious of them, you can work to control some of your unconscious eating.

Control your food cues. The best way to control your food cues is by learning to thwart them. Store fattening nibbles in out-of-sight places—at the back of the refrigerator, the backs of cabinets

Put low-fat foods up front and reachable.

and behind things. In the obvious places, put low-fat food items like fruit and cut-up vegetables or popcorn. And if your family situation allows it, don't buy tempting foods in the first place. If it's not there, you can't eat it.

Try to do all your eating at a table in the kitchen or in the dining room. Never eat in any other room and never eat standing up—like in front of the refrigerator. While you're eating, concentrate on what you're doing—not on reading, watching TV, driving or cooking. If social gatherings are your biggest cue to eating, eat something before you go so you won't be ravenous when you get there. Avoid salty snacks, which make you want to eat and drink more, and take it easy on alcohol, which tends to reduce your inhibitions about eating.

Develop new eating skills. Many people eat too much simply because they eat too fast. Experts feel that, in general, overweight people eat faster than people of normal weight. How do you learn to slow down? Try laying down your fork or spoon after each bite. And chew your food thoroughly before swallowing it. Also, be the last to start eating and the last to finish. Stall any way you can. A nice side effect of eating slowly is that you learn to savor food. Remember, if eating is to be pleasurable, it deserves your time and attention.

Put down your fork after every bite.

Another skill is learning to keep your fork on your own plate—that is, resisting the temptation to eat others' leftovers. Parents often get into this habit when their kids are young; they finish those finicky eaters' dinners.

Finally, learn something from those finicky eaters by leaving a little behind on your own plate. It may break you of compulsive plate-cleaning. And leave those big family-style bowls off the table—that's food just crying out to be eaten. Serve food directly from the stove instead. And keep your mitts off the leftovers.

Drop out of the clean-plate club.

(continued on page 98)

Stroke-Buster Cookbooks

Changing your eating style to prevent stroke and heart disease is a lot more fun when you own a few good cookbooks to guide you. As you begin cutting back the fat, salt and sugar in your recipes and adding more fish, beans, grain foods (like pasta, bread and rice), vegetables and fruits, your present cookbooks may suddenly seem sadly lacking.

Many of your favorite recipes can be adapted by decreasing the amount of sugar and salt and by substituting skim milk for whole, margarine for butter. But for new recipes and for lots of tips and hints about cooking in this new healthful manner, you may want to delve into the recent crop of "new eating" cookbooks.

What should you look for in a healthy eating cookbook? We asked Judith Benn Hurley, a culinary artist who specializes in healthy cooking and who is herself a cookbook author, what *she* looks for. "First and foremost, the recipes should sound and look delicious. No matter how much you need to change your diet, no matter if 12 doctors tell you to do so—nobody is going to prepare and eat food that doesn't taste and look good.

"Next, check to see if the recipes are really healthful. Are they really low in fat, especially saturated fat? Do they go light on salt? It's helpful if they list the percentage of calories from fat, milligrams of salt, grams of fiber and so on in each serving.

"Finally, will the recipes actually work, or are they too complicated? If they're full of ingredients that are too hard to find, you may want to think twice about it. And if they suggest you use whole wheat flour to prepare fine, light pastry, for example, steer clear—it just won't turn out," she says.

All of which suggests that you use your best instincts as a cook when evaluating cookbooks. The other thing you could do is to contact your local affiliate of the American Heart Association (AHA), to see if there's a course offered in your area on how to prepare healthy meals. Many chapters offer such a course, says Becky Lankenau, director of nutrition programs for the AHA. It's usually a six-session program, team-taught by a registered dietitian and a home economist. After taking that course, you'll be better able to evaluate cookbooks.

For now, here's a list of some of the best cookbooks available to help you prevent stroke and heart disease.

The New American Diet by Sonja L. Connor and William E. Connor, M.D. Simon & Schuster, 1986. This is much more than just a cookbook, although it's got lots of good recipes. It's loaded with tips and hints about how to change your diet gradually, from the researchers who headed the Family Heart Study, a five-year study that looked at the ability of 233 typical American families to change to healthier eating habits. After five years, 90 percent of the families were still participating, proof positive that the recipes and tips included here work.

American Heart Association Cookbook, 4th ed., David McKay Company, 1984. This also contains lots of good shopping and cooking tips for healthier eating, as well as a wide variety of recipes.

Jane Brody's Good Food Book by Jane Brody/ W. W. Norton and Company, 1985. Good hints and instructions to transform your diet into a high carbohydrate one. Lots of good information about different kinds of grains, beans, vegetables and fruits, with loads of recipes.

The Lose Weight Naturally Cookbook by Sharon Claessens and the Rodale Food Center/ Rodale Press, 1985. While the emphasis here is on losing weight, the recipes help you to do so by stressing reduced fat and increased fiber and carbohydrate foods.

Healthy Microwave Cooking by Judith Benn Hurley/Rodale Press, 1988. If you have a microwave, you'll appreciate this book's emphasis on using a microwave oven to cook foods more healthfully. Lots of good tips and recipes.

How to Find
a Stroke-Prevention
Nutritionist

Looking for a nutritionist who can help you put together the healthy eating habits we're detailing in these pages? Many doctors now recommend nutritionists to their patients with signs of cardiovascular disease that could lead to stroke or heart attack.

What should a good nutritionist be able to do for you? First and foremost, she should be able to help you plan a slow, steady attack on unhealthy eating habits by examining your present diet.

The changes should be custom-tailored and should take into account the foods you like to eat. After all, you're not going to change to a way of eating you don't like. A nutritionist should also assess your family situation and your work schedule. Do you eat away from home a lot? Does someone else prepare your food? She should also be able to give you advice on food shopping and preparation and be someone you can depend on for moral support as you make these changes.

Plan your meals in advance. Unstructured eating is the kind that usually gets out of control. Try to plan where, when and what you're going to eat. And if you do eat at an unplanned time, just remain aware that you're doing it.

Be assertive. Don't let the people around you talk you into overeating. You can politely tell the food preparer in your house what you're doing and ask for cooperation. The same goes for friends, when you're dining in restaurants or at others' homes.

Don't get discouraged and quit when you reach a plateau. There are times in every weight-loss program when you reach a plateau; that is, a

Ignore any weight-loss plateau.

The American Heart Association suggests that you choose a nutritionist who's been certified a registered dietitian by the American Dietetic Association (ADA)—you'll know because the initials "R.D." will follow her name. You may even be able to find one who specializes in working with people who have cardiovascular problems.

To find a nutritionist, check first with your doctor to see if he can refer you. If you don't have any luck there, check with the AHA affiliate in your area. You could also check with your local hospital or look in your phone book under "Dietitians" or "Nutritionists." Or, if there's a university nearby, check with its nutrition department.

The ADA will send you a list of its consulting member dietitians for your state if you send a stamped, self-addressed envelope. Write to the American Dietetic Association, 208 South LaSalle Street, Chicago, IL 60604-1003, Attention: Division of Practice.

The cost for nutrition services is sometimes covered by medical insurance if you've been referred by a physician, so be sure to get a referral if you can.

time when, despite your best efforts, you don't seem to be losing weight. Don't let it throw you. Forget about watching the scale and instead focus on your successes—you've really changed your eating habits permanently to a low-fat diet, for example, or you're regularly exercising four times a week. Concentrating on your successes can really get you over the "plateau" hurdle. And soon the pounds will start falling off again—seemingly on their own.

Keep your weight-loss program fun. Learn delicious new low-fat recipes and have fun preparing and eating them. Exercise with a friend if you hate exercising alone. Remember, you're not going

Go easy on yourself.

to stick to a program you hate.

Don't feel like a failure if you overeat. Many people get so disgusted with themselves that they abandon all efforts to control their eating after one indiscretion. Instead, go easy on yourself. Tell yourself that next time you'll do better. And keep thinking positively about all the strides you've already made.

Besides these techniques, there's one other surefire way to help yourself lose weight—physical activity. And that's what the next chapter is all about.

Chapter 5

Exercise: The One-Two Punch against Stroke

Remember that feeling you used to have when you were seven, after a brisk afternoon of running around, jumping in leaves, climbing up trees and riding your bicycle? Your blood raced, your lungs were full, your heart pounded. Becoming active again, this time as an adult, is like a joyous return to that bursting-with-life feeling. And that alone should be temptation enough to lure you back into the world of physical fitness.

But if it isn't—then sit back for a minute. We've got an avalanche of other reasons—all of which tie in perfectly with your stroke-prevention program—that you should jump out of your chair after reading this and lace up your sneakers again.

Let's begin at the most important point—exercise's contribution to preventing cardiovascular disease, the disease that causes most strokes and heart attacks. How do scientists know that exercise has a positive effect? Mostly by studying the health habits of large groups of people and then

Lace up your sneakers.

keeping track to see which of them develop cardio-vascular problems.

One such study, performed at the University of North Carolina at Chapel Hill, used precise treadmill tests to measure the fitness levels of over 3,000 healthy men aged 30 through 69. Eight years later, the researchers looked at those same men again and found that the ones with the lowest fitness ratings had a 3.4 times greater risk of dying of a stroke or a heart attack than men with the highest fitness ratings. In fact, being in the lowest fitness group was an even greater risk than being a smoker.

Another massive study of almost 17,000 Harvard alumni found that physical activity—walking, stair climbing, sports, anything that burned extra calories and raised the pulse rate—kept the men who were active alive longer, especially protecting them from cardiovascular and respiratory disease.

And as researchers zero in on stroke risk, the protective effect of exercise still stands. In the Netherlands, for example, a team of researchers followed an entire community for several years, monitoring people of all ages for the appearance of virtually all the stroke risk factors. The results showed that people who engaged in regular exercise—light or heavy—had only 40 percent the stroke risk of the rest of that Dutch community who just sat around.

But exercise's benefits don't stop there. When you look at individual stroke risk factors, there are additional good effects. "I'm beginning to wonder if the disease we call hypertension [high blood pressure] isn't in fact due to a lifestyle in which we don't exercise as we should," says professor of medicine Robert Cade, M.D., of the University of Florida at Gainesville. Dr. Cade has studied the effects of aerobic exercise on over 400 people. He found that blood pressure went down in 96 *percent* of them. And that was the result of their taking walks just three to five times a week.

A lack of exercise may be riskier than smoking.

Regular exercise lowered stroke risk by 60 percent in one community.

Other studies have confirmed exercise's downward effect on high blood pressure, which is the most potent risk factor for stroke. With just 45 minutes of bicycling three times a week, people with hypertension enjoyed impressive reductions in their blood pressure readings, according to an Australian study. And these people made no other changes in their lifestyles or diets (studies have shown that losing weight and cutting back on salt and alcohol can also bring down high blood pressure).

Forty-five minutes of bicycling three times a week also lowered blood pressure.

Moreover, when researchers looked at the blood pressures of the Harvard alumni mentioned earlier, they found that those who did not exercise were 35 percent more likely to develop high blood pressure later in life. That tendency remained whether or not they were overweight or had a family history of high blood pressure, both of which further increase the risk of getting the disease.

And in another 12-year-long study of more than 6,000 men and women, those who had low levels of physical fitness at the beginning of the study were half again as likely to develop high blood pressure as their counterparts who were fitter. That was regardless of their age, sex, weight and blood pressure at the beginning of the study— all of which could affect their later tendency to develop high blood pressure. (The fact that extra weight has been linked to high blood pressure, however, is an added argument for staying active, since exercise helps most people lose weight. More on that later.)

Couch potatoes are 50 percent more likely to develop high blood pressure.

A third reason exercise may reduce your risk of having a stroke or heart attack is that it goes after another potent risk factor: high blood cholesterol. Kenneth Cooper, M.D., the doctor who coined the term *aerobics*, reports that data from more than 18,000 people who've been tested at his research facilities shows that the greater their levels of physical fitness, the lower their total blood cholesterol levels. He also found that fitter people had

The higher your level of fitness, the lower your level of cholesterol.

higher levels of HDL cholesterol, the "good" cholesterol that helps clear your arteries of fatty deposits.

Even among people with heart disease who came to the Cooper Clinic, those who exercised and became fitter enjoyed an increase in their HDL levels, reported Dr. Cooper at a cholesterol conference held at his Institute for Aerobics Research in Dallas.

Exercise knocks out blood clots.

But besides keeping cholesterol at healthy levels, exercise does other good things for your blood. Studies have shown that it helps prevent the formation of dangerous blood clots, which can lodge in an artery supplying blood to your brain, causing a stroke. Finnish researchers recently found, for example, that after a 12-week exercise program, men who worked out were much less likely to experience dangerous clots than another group that didn't exercise.

Exercise may be the ultimate "diet."

Exercise is also a powerful way to lose weight—and that can reduce your risk of developing high blood pressure, high cholesterol and diabetes—all stroke risk factors. Is it really possible to use exercise as your weight-loss method? Yes; in fact, it's superior to dieting alone because exercise burns off fat while dieting tends to make you lose muscle as well as fat.

How do we know? Well one study, for example, looked at a group of women who checked into a weight-loss clinic after countless attempts to shed pounds. Instead of putting them on yet another diet, doctors at the clinic decided to try a different approach—exercise. The women were told to exercise at least 30 minutes a day. All chose walking. And the more the women walked, the more weight they lost, from 10 to 38 pounds the first year.

Most important, as long as the women kept up their walking programs, they never regained any weight. And they did it all without changing their eating habits.

Why is exercise such an efficient way to lose weight? Experts believe that exercise gives your metabolism a boost. After you exercise, you may burn calories more efficiently for up to 24 hours— even while you sleep! Exercise can also stimulate your body to generate more heat, which also helps burn calories. And exercise can keep your appetite in check.

> Exercise boosts your metabolism—even while you sleep.

How? The energy used by your body during exercise is released into your bloodstream as glucose, a form of sugar. Your appetite regulator, the hypothalamus, recognizes higher blood sugar levels and remains satisfied longer before signaling hunger. Low blood sugar levels, on the other hand, also trigger the hypothalamus—to make you hungry.

Hungry for more information on how to get in shape? Let's begin.

On Your Mark . . .

You've probably noticed that the kind of exercises performed by people in the studies we've cited is the kind that gets you up out of your chair and moving at a continuous pace. Walking, jogging, bicycling, swimming and dancing are probably the best examples of this kind of exercise, which the experts call "aerobic."

Aerobic exercise is the kind that benefits your cardiovascular system the most because it makes your heart stronger and improves blood circulation. It's also the form of exercise that lowers your blood pressure and blood cholesterol and helps regulate your weight and blood sugar.

> "Aerobic" exercise strengthens your heart.

Exercises like weight training, calisthenics and stretching make your muscles stronger and more supple, which will help you exercise more efficiently and protect you from injuries, but they generally don't do a lot to improve your cardiovascular system. They should be done as a complement to aerobic exercise, never in place of it.

How do you know you're getting an aerobic workout? "You should move to the point where you can continue talking, but you're huffing and puffing a bit," says Ron Lawrence, M.D., a California neurologist who is head of the American Medical Athletic Association. "Also, you should work up a low-grade perspiration and be moving the large muscles in your arms and legs in a continuous, rhythmic fashion."

Exercise experts have come up with a scientific way of measuring this state as a way of checking whether you're exercising strenuously enough to get an aerobic workout. It's a way of estimating how hard your heart is working to accomplish your physical goals. It's also a way to check yourself to be sure you're not overstressing your heart. That's why many doctors recommend that you learn it.

You measure how hard your heart is working by learning to count the number of times your heart beats per minute. That's your heart rate. At rest, the average heart beats about 72 times per minute (although you can be well above or below that figure and still be considered normal).

When you exercise, your heart starts to beat faster, up to a level that exercise physiologists call your "maximum heart rate." You don't have to work up to that level to get aerobic benefits, however. In fact, for safety's sake, you shouldn't. You can achieve cardiovascular fitness by working at an exercise intensity that's between 60 and 80 percent of it—a figure called your "target heart rate."

How do you determine your target heart rate? The simplest way is to begin by finding your maximum heart rate, which is done by subtracting your age from the number 220. A 40-year-old's maximum heart rate, for example, would be 180. Forty from 220 is 180, right? Then the same 40-year-old would calculate his *target* heart rate by figuring out that 60 and 80 percent of 180 are 108 and 144. That means he should exercise up to a heart rate of between 108 and 144 beats per minute. (If you don't feel like doing the math, see the table, "Find Your Target Heart Rate," on page 107 for the target heart rates for people between 20 and 70.)

How do you keep an eye on your heart rate? The easiest way is to place a finger—not your thumb since it has its own pulse—on the pulse at your wrist. Count the number of beats in 10 seconds and then multiply by 6—that's your heart rate, the number of times your heart is beating per minute. You should take your pulse several times during any exercise session to be sure your heart rate is in the target range.

How often and how long do you need to exercise to prevent strokes? The American College of Sports Medicine recommends that you exercise regularly, about three times a week, or every other day, to benefit your cardiovascular system. You should keep your heart rate in the target area for about 30 to 45 minutes at each session, depending on how strenuous the exercise is. A fast runner, for example, wouldn't need to exercise as long as a brisk walker to get the same benefits.

You need to exercise three times a week to do your cardiovascular system any good.

Find Your Target Heart Rate

To find your target heart rate, look up your age range on the left. Then look to the right of those numbers to find the range of heartbeats per minute you should maintain while exercising. Beginning exercisers should stick to 60 percent of their maximum heart rate, while more experienced exercisers can go up to 70 and 80 percent of their maximum.

Age	Target Heart Rate (beats per minute)		
	60%	70%	80%
20–29	114–120	134–140	153–160
30–39	109–114	127–133	145–152
40–49	103–108	120–126	137–144
50–59	97–102	113–119	129–136
60–69	91–96	106–112	121–128

SOURCE: *Official YMCA Fitness Program*, National Board of YMCAs (Rosemont, Ill: National Board of YMCAs, 1984).

Get Set . . .

Before you start any exercise program, you should always check with your doctor, especially if you are over 35. He will give you a physical and perhaps run an exercise stress test—an electrocardiogram while you are stressing your heart through physical activity.

Check out your body.

The most well-known method is while you walk on a treadmill. The electrocardiogram machine, which records your heartbeat and heart rhythm, will tell your doctor how your heart functions under physical stress, particularly whether or not it's getting enough oxygen as you exercise. If it's not, that's a key indication that the arteries supplying blood to your heart are clogged or blocked, which means you may be suffering from atherosclerosis and cardiovascular disease.

But that doesn't mean you should forget about exercising. If anything, that's usually the opposite of what you should do, says George Sheehan, M.D., a cardiologist, runner, popular speaker and author. The results of a stress test will help your doctor prescribe an exercise program that is safe for you, given your individual circumstances.

Find your comfort zone.

"You'll have to exercise within a comfort zone, that is, with no pain," says Dr. Sheehan. And your doctor will probably want you to work on eliminating some other controllable risk factors for cardiovascular disease, such as reducing cholesterol levels or losing weight. If so, exercise is still your best bet for doing that, believes Dr. Sheehan.

Whatever the state of your cardiovascular health, be sure to begin exercising safely. Go slowly for the first three to four weeks, especially if you are over 50 or haven't exercised before, advises the American Medical Athletic Association's Dr. Lawrence. Once you've grown accustomed to movement, aim for a target heart rate at the lower end of the range—60 percent of your maximum heart rate is enough to enjoy cardiovascular benefits, he says. You can stay at that level and continue to benefit, although many people like to challenge themselves by progressing to higher levels. That's fine if your body can tolerate it.

"What you want to aim for is a state of good health, where your cardiovascular and respiratory system can take sustained physical activity for a period of time," says Dr. Lawrence. "Your heart rate should recover and go back to normal quickly after you exercise, and you should have no difficulty breathing while you're exercising."

Go!

To avoid injuring your muscles or overtaxing your heart, be sure to warm up adequately before you begin exercising. Loosen your muscles with some easy walking or light jogging in place. This begins to warm up your muscles and prepare them for more intense activity. Then do a few simple stretching exercises and begin your exercise activity slowly, picking up speed until you're up to your target heart rate.

Warm-ups avoid burn-ups.

And with that thought in mind, here's a rundown on some of the most popular forms of exercise that can give you cardiovascular benefits.

Walk Away from Stroke

New scientific research—and a lot of it—focuses on walking's benefits as an aerobic exercise that can improve your cardiovascular health and prevent stroke. In fact, researchers are finding that walking can hold its own when pitted against more vigorous kinds of aerobic exercise, like jogging.

Walking is where stroke prevention begins.

According to studies performed at Stanford University School of Medicine, brisk walking can reduce your risk of cardiovascular disease about 80 percent as effectively as jogging.

**Walking lowers your
blood pressure.**

Walking has also been successfully used to help people keep their blood pressures down and their levels of HDL cholesterol (the good kind) up. And no section about walking would be complete without mentioning its slow but steady ability to help you lose weight. This is worth mentioning because many people don't think walking is vigorous enough exercise to burn calories. (See the table, "How Many Calories in a Mile?" below.) But it is. You just need to adjust your expectations of how fast you'll lose weight, because it takes longer to achieve your goals.

Weight loss by walking is best thought about over a period of months, not days. Set your sights on six months or a year from now, not six days. Here's an example of that kind of thinking.

Say you walk at an easy to moderate pace for 40 minutes. At a rate of about 20 minutes to the mile, you'll have walked 2 miles. If you weigh 140, your total calories burned would be $2 \times 95 = 190$.

How Many Calories in a Mile?

Add up the calories you burn by walking. A typical 3-mile walk for a 150-pound person, for example, would use up 300 calories. Do that three or four times a week and you're on the slow, sure path to weight loss.

Weight	Approximate Calorie Burn per Mile
120	80
130	87
140	95
150	100
160	105
170	111
180	115
190	120
200	123

Do that every day for 30 days and you've walked away $30 \times 190 = 5{,}700$ calories. Since there are 3,500 calories in a pound, you've just walked off a pound and a half. Do it for six months and you'll have lost 9 pounds. And that's without restricting your food intake at all!

Keep in mind that weight-loss experts say this slow path is your best guarantee that lost pounds will stay lost. It gives your body and appetite time to adjust to the lower weight, and it allows you to keep up a healthy, nutritious diet. Most important, the pounds you'll be losing will be all fat. People who lose weight by dieting alone lose both muscle *and* fat.

When you walk off the pounds, they stay gone.

But perhaps the most compelling argument for making a good walk the centerpiece of your fitness program is that you're much more likely to stick to it than to other forms of exercise. It's easier. You don't need to change your clothes except to lace on a good pair of walking shoes. You don't need to travel to a health club. And you can weave it into your daily routine by walking to do errands, catch a bus, even entertain your kids.

Why is stick-to-itiveness an important factor in an exercise program? Well, all those marvelous benefits we've cited above happen only to people who exercise regularly. If you choose an exercise that you don't feel comfortable doing or one that you can't seem to fit into your lifestyle, you're probably going to quit before long—no matter how much money you've spent on clothes or a club membership.

Fit your exercise into your lifestyle.

So having considered all that, how do you get started? Before you set foot to road, step into a comfortable pair of shoes. If you already own a pair of sneakers or running shoes, they should do fine. Experts agree that any shoe that provides basic comfort and stability can make for a safe and enjoyable journey.

If you don't own a pair of exercise shoes, check out the incredible variety of walking shoes

Make your feet feel comfortable.

crowding the shelves. These represent the shoe industry's best efforts to make our feet feel comfortable. Look for a well-cushioned, even "springy" heel, sturdy construction and above all, a comfortable fit. A shoe that will also control but not eliminate the tendency of your foot to roll inward is also a good idea.

Once your feet are comfortable, it's time to decide on a plan of action to launch your walking program. You'll want to work in at least 30 minutes of brisk walking three times a week, says Barry Franklin, Ph.D., director of the Cardiac Rehabilitation Laboratories at William Beaumont Hospital in Royal Oak, Michigan. Even better would be to walk 45 to 60 minutes four days a week.

Walk at least three times a week.

What does brisk mean? Dr. Franklin pegs it at about 4 miles an hour, or 15 minutes to the mile. Of course, you won't do that your first day out—and you shouldn't. Walking, like any other physical activity, should be approached gradually.

One easy way to do this—and one that will motivate you as well—is to regard your first 15-minute mile as a goal to work toward, like an Olympic athlete trains to break a new mileage record. When you achieve that goal, your feeling of accomplishment should spur you on to bigger and better things, says Robert S. Brown, M.D., Ph.D., a professor of behavioral medicine and psychiatry at the University of Virginia in Charlottesville. Here's Dr. Brown's plan of action:

Set yourself a goal.

Measure out a 1-mile course.

Measure out a 1-mile course by using your car's odometer. Or find a track you can use. (Indoor tracks are usually ⅛ or 1⁄16 mile, outdoor tracks ¼ mile.) Walk the course at a pace you can easily tolerate and check to see how long it takes you. Stop if you feel short of breath or experience pain. Walk the same course each day while keeping track of your time. When you can comfortably walk the course in 15 minutes, you will have broken the 15-minute barrier. Congratulations! Give yourself a well-deserved pat on the back.

Now work toward your *next* goal: to walk 2 miles in 30 minutes. Gradually increase to 2 miles. Once you've reached that goal—you've won again. Now it's on to 3 miles in 45 minutes, using the same methods. Before you know it, you'll be filling Dr. Franklin's prescription of a 45- to 60-minute brisk walk. Now, if you can plan to do that every other day or four days a week, you've made it as a fitness walker. Keep up the good work.

If you find it harder than you imagined it would be to keep up the pace of a good walking program, however, you may want to check your walking style. Although it seems like the easiest job around, there really is a "technique" to this kind of walking.

Are you breathing deeply and rhythmically? If you're not, you could feel more winded and tired than you need to. With every five or six steps, inhale deeply, hold the breath for a few steps and then exhale slowly.

Learn how to breathe.

Is your body straight? Many people walk with their upper body falling forward, letting their legs catch up. Instead, your body should be straight, with your legs leading the way.

Are you walking with a full stride? Don't take short steps or bend your knees a lot.

Are you walking rhythmically? An erratic walking pace can tire you out. Instead, walk with a steady cadence.

One of the great things about a regular walking program, as we mentioned earlier, is that it fits into all settings in a quick, no-frills way. But if you're finding it hard to make the time for walking, here are a few suggestions.

Work walking into your life.

Walk part of your commute. If you take a train or bus to work, get off one station or stop sooner on the way to work and board one station or stop later on the way home.

Walk at the beginning or end of your work-day. Avoid the crowds at peak commuting times and leave early for work, then walk before the workday begins. Or take a walk after work, before beginning your commute home.

Discover the 3-mile lunch. When you're planning a business meeting at the lunch hour, organize it around a brisk walk. That is, get the walk in first and pick up a quick lunch afterward.

Walk your errands instead of driving them. Do you need to make a stop at the dry cleaner, the pet store and the bank? Patronize stores that are relatively close together and walk your errands. You'll save yourself the aggravation of traffic and parking, too.

Avoid vacation trouble.

Plan a walking vacation. Many people gain weight on vacation by sitting on tour buses or spending all their time in the car. Since most of us eat more when we're traveling, that can mean double trouble. Instead, plan a vacation where you explore a city by foot (many local chambers of commerce have developed walking tours to help you out). Or make a trip to the mountains or a state park, where there's plenty of opportunity for nature walks.

But, although you can't beat walking for its safety, ease and ability to fit into almost any schedule, there are also other great aerobic exercises you may be interested in trying. Here's a quick run-down.

Run for Your Life

Try a run on the open road.

If your heart thrills just a little when you see TV footage of the men and women breaking the ribbon as they win the Boston or New York marathon, or if the thought of donning a jogging suit and taking to the open road appeals to you, then you may want to give running or jogging a try. Approached slowly and maintained safely, a running program is a great way to stay physically fit. And it doesn't take as much time as walking.

The downside of running is that you run a greater risk of getting injured—especially in your knees, legs and feet, says Bryant Stamford, Ph.D., an exercise physiologist who is director of the health promotion and wellness program at the University of Louisville, Kentucky.

But to keep injuries at bay, it's important to warm up before a run and not push yourself beyond safe distances. Aerobics expert Dr. Kenneth Cooper says a safe running program—one that will help prevent injuries while yielding cardiovascular benefits—involves running 20 to 30 minutes a session, four times a week. The maximum number of miles he recommends is 12 to 15 per week.

Go for 20- to 30-minute runs four times a week.

You can also protect yourself from running injuries by exercising late in the day. One study found that the greatest number of injuries occurred in morning runners, the least in afternoon runners. The doctors who conducted the study thought at the time that this might be because muscle tissue is well-stretched later in the day, making it more flexible and less vulnerable to injury.

Afternoon runs are less likely to result in injuries.

A second study of runners' injuries—in this case knee injuries—found that problems were more likely to occur in runners who had increased their mileage or speed too quickly, or abruptly changed from one running surface to another—from grass during the summer, for example, to an indoor track in the winter.

And, finally, running shoes that are poorly made or just badly fitted can cause injuries, too. So it pays to invest in a good pair before starting your running program, advises John W. Pagliano, D.P.M., a Long Beach, California, podiatrist who evaluates running shoes. Look for a shoe that is built to absorb the shock of pounding on a hard surface, with a lot of support in the heel area to keep your foot from rolling in or out—a motion that can cause injuries to your foot, lower leg and knee.

How to begin a running program? It's best to start by working up to a brisk walking program first, says Dr. Stamford. Once you can do that easily, begin a second phase by jogging for short intervals while you continue to mostly walk. Phase three would have you walking and jogging in about equal amounts. In the fourth phase you'd begin to do more jogging than walking, and the final phase would be all jogging. Spend about two to three weeks in each phase, Dr. Stamford advises, before moving on to the next.

A four-step program to get your started.

For Stroke Prevention—Stroke

Running leaves you more vulnerable to injuries than any other aerobic exercise; swimming is its exact opposite. In fact, many experts call swimming the *perfect* exercise: Since your weight is supported when you swim, you get an aerobic workout that strengthens your muscles and keeps them flexible with a minimum risk of injury.

Swimming may be the best exercise.

And swimming can increase your cardiovascular fitness as effectively as walking and running, as a study of middle-aged people at the University of Texas Health Science Center in Dallas indicated. The study found that after a 12-week program of intense training in the pool, the hearts of participants worked better. Quite simply, they had the capacity to pump more blood.

But with all these pluses, it's still important to keep in mind the minuses of swimming, says Dr. Stamford. "Swimming is tough to do if you've never developed the skill before. To swim laps, you have to learn the various strokes, and that takes time," he points out. Also, there's the convenience factor. Do you have a pool nearby that's accessible and suitable for swimming laps? A recreational pool with millions of kids splashing around won't leave much room for serious swim-

A Walk/Jog Program for the Weekend Athlete

Maybe you're the kind of person who just can't fit exercise into the busy workweek. Maybe you just don't like exercising enough to make an every-other-day commitment. Or maybe you're an occasional tennis player, golfer or recreational exerciser who'd like to put a little extra time into improving your cardiovascular fitness.

If you fit any of these descriptions, this weekend fitness program is for you. You won't lose a lot of weight or be able to run a marathon on this program, but you'll be a lot better off than someone who is completely sedentary.

This walk/jog program is designed to increase your fitness levels gradually over three to five months, according to Bryant Stamford, Ph.D., an exercise physiologist who put together the program.

Why so slow? "People who embark on a weekend exercise program have to realize that their progress must be slower than that of a more regular exerciser," says Dr. Stamford, who is director of the health promotion program at the University of Louisville, Kentucky. This gradual buildup won't overstress your joints and you'll also avoid the aches and pains that often cause weekend athletes to give up quickly.

The walk/jog program begins by helping you build distance. You begin with half a mile, then increase a quarter mile each weekend. Once you've hit 3 miles, it works on increasing intensity, which Dr. Stamford describes as the ratio of walking paces to jogging paces. You'll notice that the intensity is different for people under 35 and for people over 35. If you're over 35, you'll be increasing intensity a little more slowly. "Once you've mastered both distance and intensity," says Dr. Stamford, "you'll be doing the kind of workout you can easily maintain for the rest of your life."

Weekend	Miles per Session	Intensity per Session			
		Under Age 35		Over Age 35	
		Walking Paces	Jogging Paces	Walking Paces	Jogging Paces
1	½	50	50	75	25
2	¾	50	50	75	25
3	1	50	50	75	25
4	1¼	50	50	75	25
5	1½	50	50	75	25
6	1¾	50	50	75	25
7	2	50	50	75	25
8	2¼	50	50	75	25
9	2½	50	50	75	25
10	2¾	50	50	75	25
11	3	50	50	75	25

(continued)

A Walk/Jog Program for the Weekend Athlete—Continued

Weekend	Miles per Session	Intensity per Session			
		Under Age 35		Over Age 35	
		Walking Paces	Jogging Paces	Walking Paces	Jogging Paces
12	3	50	100	50	50
13	3	50	200	50	70
14	3	all jog		50	90
15	3	all jog		50	110
16	3	all jog		50	130
17	3	all jog		50	150
18	3	all jog		50	170
19	3	all jog		50	190
20	3	all jog		all jog	

SOURCE: Bryant Stamford, Ph.D., Health Promotion Program, University of Louisville School of Medicine.

NOTE: If you're not at all active when starting this program, Dr. Stamford recommends slowing down the intensity buildup by half. In other words, the under-35 athlete would increase the jog paces by only 25 per weekend (starting at the 12th weekend), instead of 50, until he's up to 200 jog paces. The over-35 athlete would increase the jog paces by only 10 per weekend (starting at the 13th weekend) instead of 20.

Alternate swimming and resting to get started.

ming. And do you have the time in your schedule to shower, dress and dry your hair afterward?

If you have the time and a convenient location and swimming is the exercise you most enjoy, then by all means go to it! Refamiliarize yourself with the various strokes and practice your form to begin with, says Dr. Stamford. Then get into swimming laps gradually by alternating between swimming and resting until you've built up your endurance.

What's the best swimming stroke to strengthen your cardiovascular system? It's really better to know and use a variety of strokes, believes Jane Katz, Ed.D., a professor of health and physical education and the author of several books on swimming for fitness. That way, you'll use a variety of muscles and add diversity to your workouts—which can keep you motivated.

Having said that, however, it's also useful to know how the various strokes rate according to their strenuousness. (The more strenuous they are, the better able you may be to keep your heart rate at an aerobically beneficial level. Of course, if you're out of shape, then any of the strokes will probably get your heart pumping). Here's Dr. Katz's rating, from the most to the least strenuous.

The crawl. Also called freestyle, this stroke is not only the most strenuous and the fastest, it's also the easiest to learn for most people, says Dr. Katz. That's because the arm and leg movements are similar to those of walking. The crawl uses about 20 percent leg movement and 80 percent arm movement. It's great for toning up the muscles in your upper arms and shoulders, as well as your front thigh and calf muscles.

The backstroke. This is the second most strenuous and the second fastest stroke. Its big disadvantage is that it's difficult for you to see where you're going—a problem if you're swimming laps in a crowded pool. The backstroke uses about 25 percent leg power and 75 percent arm power. It uses the same muscles as the crawl, as well as giving your chest muscles a good workout.

The breaststroke. Largely due to its long, restful glide motion, the breaststroke is a tad less strenuous than the crawl and the backstroke, says Dr. Katz. However, it's great to do in rough water, a busy pool or any other situation where you're likely to encounter obstacles, because you have excellent visibility. The breaststroke uses about 50 percent leg power and 50 percent arm power to get you through the water. It's also a good exercise to tone your inner and outer thighs, inner and upper arms and chest muscles.

Use a variety of strokes.

Give your chest muscles a good workout with the backstroke.

The sidestroke. This is probably the least effective stroke for improving your physical fitness, says Dr. Katz, but it's great to use when you want to vary your pace or you don't feel up to a more strenuous swim. The sidestroke uses about 50 percent leg power and about 50 percent arm power. It's a good exercise for your inner leg muscles and the muscles in your sides.

If you use swimming as your aerobic activity, you should know that your heart rate naturally stays somewhat lower than when you're doing other aerobic exercises. It's due to the "diving reflex," a natural lowering of heart rate that occurs just by putting your face in the water. Experts think it happens for several reasons. For one thing, you breathe differently when swimming than during landlubbing activities. Also, the lying-down position you're in while swimming enables the heart to pump more blood with each beat, so it doesn't have to work as hard.

That's why you shouldn't expect your heart rate to rise quite as high when you swim. If you want to figure out your target heart rate for swimming, subtract your age from 205 rather than 220, advises William McArdle, Ph.D., an exercise physiologist from Queens College, New York, who has researched swimming and heart rate. Then find 60 to 80 percent of that figure to use as your target heart rate range.

If you're not interested in swimming laps, but you love the water or are injury-prone, you might want to try out a water aerobics class. Offered now at many health clubs, spas and YMCAs (Young Men's Christian Association), the classes are usually set to music and include calistheniclike routines and jogging in the water.

"You can do all kinds of creative exercises that will raise your heart rate while you're working against the resistance of water," says Dr. Stamford. There are also several books on the market filled

Just putting your face in the water will lower your heart rate.

A quick way to calculate your target heart rate for swimming.

with water exercise routines, so check your local bookstore if there are no classes in your area.

Pedal Away from Strokes

Although outdoor cycling is a good complement to a general fitness program—and can be very challenging if you meet up with some inclines and hills—it's generally not challenging enough to give your heart a truly superior aerobic workout, says Dr. Stamford. That's not to say you should give up cycling if it's a favorite activity. Just monitor your heart rate and try to keep the workout strenuous. Dr. Cooper has found that while speeds of less than 10 miles per hour are generally not worth much aerobically for the average person, a speed of slightly greater than 15 miles per hour will give you a good workout.

Cycling at speeds of more than 15 miles per hour will give you a good workout.

Of course, you won't start out at that rate. Ease into a biking program slowly, especially if you're over 40, says Dr. Lawrence. (See the table, "A Beginner's Cycling Program," on page 122.) Cycling's greatest benefit is that, like swimming, it's a nonweight-bearing activity, so you're less vulnerable to injury.

Cycling gives you exercise without weight stress.

If you like the idea of cycling for aerobic exercise, you may want to try indoor cycling on a stationary bicycle—the most popular piece of exercise equipment on the market. This method of wheel spinning gives you a great workout, since you're able to set the resistance of the bike high enough to raise your heart rate to aerobic levels, says Dr. Stamford.

Try a stationary bike.

But before you choose an exercise bike for your home, be sure to give the bike a 15-minute test, suggest John Krausz and Vera van der Ries Krausz, bicycling experts and authors of a book on stationary biking. Grip the seat firmly with two hands and try to move it up and down. It shouldn't tilt or shift forward or back. If it does, you'll risk slipping or falling during your ride. Next, sit on the bike. Is the seat high enough so you can extend one leg straight down (with the knee flexed, not locked)? If not, can the seat be

A Beginner's Cycling Program

This cycling program is suggested by Ron Lawrence, M.D., for people over 40 who are beginning to use a bicycle for fitness riding. You'll notice that some weeks you increase your mileage, while other weeks you increase your speed. If the schedule is too vigorous for you, just repeat a week. Plan to ride at least three days a week; four would be even better. When you reach 23 weeks, keep riding at the speed and mileage indicated until it gets too easy. Then increase your mileage gradually until you're riding an hour at each session.

Week	Miles	Minutes	Miles per Hour
1	at your ease	at your ease	at your ease
2	1 or 2	at your ease	at your ease
3	3	18	10
4	4	24	10
5	4	20	12
6	4	18	13.5
7	4	16	15
8	5	30	10
9	5	25	12
10	5	22	13.5
11	5	20	15
12	6	36	10
13	6	30	12
14	6	27	13.5
15	6	24	15
16	7	42	10
17	7	35	12
18	7	31	13.5
19	7	28	15
20	8	48	10
21	8	40	12
22	8	35	13.5
23	8	32	15

SOURCE: Adapted from *Going the Distance*, Ron Lawrence and Sandra Rosenzweig (New York: Tarcher/St. Martin's Press, 1987).

adjusted so you can? Are the handlebars adjustable so you can reach them without effort? This can make your ride more comfortable, too.

Now pedal backward. A too-high seat will cause your hips to rock back and forth. See if you can adjust the seat to prevent that from happening.

Start a 10-minute ride pedaling forward. Look down over the wheel as you ride. It should be perfectly centered and wobble-free. (The bike should have a centering adjustment for the wheel.) Now try to gauge the comfort of the seat. Would you prefer a wider or narrower one? Do you need more padding to avoid getting sore? If you can't find a seat that suits you on any bike you try, don't despair. Most bicycling shops sell seats in a variety of sizes with posts to fit stationary bikes. So if you've found the perfect bike except for the seat, you can always adapt that later.

Take a trial ride.

Machines that Can Help

Along with exercise bikes, rowing machines and treadmills can give you an effective aerobic workout in the warmth and comfort of your home or at a health club. If you're thinking of buying either of these machines, here's a quick rundown on what to watch for.

Rowing machines. Look for a smooth seat action with no jitters. Rowers have sliding seats so that your legs can get in on the action. The seat should be comfortable and well-padded and you should be able to fully extend your legs during the rowing action. Also the frame should be solid enough so that the machine doesn't jump around the floor every time you row back and forth. Be sure you can adjust the resistance on the rower so you can challenge yourself enough to get a good workout.

Rowing machines and treadmills allow you to work out at home.

Treadmills. These come in motorized and nonmotorized versions. Although nonmotorized treadmills are much less expensive and won't usually break down, a motorized treadmill helps you maintain a steady pace for a better workout.

On motorized treadmills, look for a quiet motor, an adjustable speed control (which has a speed slow enough so that you can start out walking), and an emergency on/off switch that's easy to reach in case you need it. Front and side rails are a help to aid your balance.

Nonmotorized treadmills should have belts that move freely and without friction. The belt surface should be comfortable and well-padded, with a smooth, quiet ride. Timers and odometers are great to have on both kinds of treadmills so you can measure your workout.

Dance toward Health

Want to get aerobic benefits while enjoying your workout with a group of fellow exercisers? Then an aerobic dance class may be just the ticket. It's fun, seldom boring, and best of all, it's set to music, which can enhance your performance and help you get rid of tension. Many studies have now shown that aerobic dancing can improve your cardiovascular fitness while helping to lower your cholesterol and your weight. And perhaps most important, these studies indicate, the classes are usually so much fun that people tend to stick with them.

But, like other weight-bearing exercises, aerobic dancing has its downside. The pounding your joints and muscles take leaves you vulnerable to injury. So, like running, aerobic dance is best approached slowly. Don't try to do too much, too soon. Start by just doing a few minutes of the heavy aerobic portion of the class and then build up gradually to about a maximum of 20 minutes—that's enough to get your heart working.

Two other culprits that cause aerobic dance injuries are hard floors and poor footwear, says

Edward C. Percy, M.D., an orthopedic surgeon who specializes in sports medicine. Look for a dance surface that's cushioned—but not too soft, he says. "The surface should be cushioned enough so that there is some give, but it shouldn't be so soft that the foot sinks into it."

Hard floors and poor footwear are double trouble.

Choose aerobic shoes that are light and flexible, with a softly cushioned sole, a slightly built-up heel and a flexible toe area that will bend with your movements. The heel cup (the area that hugs your heel) should provide both cushioning and good support for your whole heel area, says Dr. Percy.

Another good way to avoid injuries is to join one of the new low-impact aerobics classes cropping up across the country. These classes replace jumping and jogging movements with marches and other moves that keep one foot on the floor at all times. This eliminates a lot of the jarring impact that makes aerobics so hard on the knees, shins and feet. Instructors are also careful to help participants stretch muscles and not force their bodies into any overextended positions. And the classes also strive to keep your heart rate at the bottom end of your target range, for heart safety's sake.

Low-impact aerobics gives you a workout without bone-jarring stress.

Start but Don't Stop

What other aerobic activities can you do? Well, if you happen to live in a part of the country where cross-country skiing is a part of your life, consider yourself very lucky. It's the most aerobically challenging sport you can practice. If you live near a resort that offers cross-country ski trails, inquire about lessons if you want to learn the sport. Most resorts will let you rent the equipment you need and guide you while you're learning.

Tennis, on the other hand, is only as aerobic as you make it. The stop-and-start nature of the activity is the problem. If you want to get aerobic benefits, play at a high enough pitch to keep your heart pumping, advises Dr. Cooper. It's better to consider tennis an alternate aerobic activity instead of the centerpiece of your fitness program.

Other racquet sports like racquetball and squash can definitely be aerobically challenging, studies show—but they're still stop-and-start activities. These should also be only a part of your total fitness regimen.

Stop-and-start sports should not be the centerpiece of your exercise program.

Winding Down

When you've finished exercising, don't just come to an abrupt halt and head for the showers. Just as you've built up your heart rate slowly, you should also bring it back down gradually, by cooling down with a less-strenuous version of the exercise you just performed. Swimmers might swim slowly for a few minutes. Joggers and fast walkers should slow down to an easy walk. Your heart needs time to recover from its exertion—if you stop too abruptly, you might put an undue strain on your whole cardiovascular system.

A cool-down keeps blood moving to your heart and brain.

Also, when you're exercising, blood collects in your arms and legs to give your limbs the nutrients and oxygen they need, says Jack Wilmore, Ph.D., former director of the Exercise and Sports Sciences Laboratory at the University of Arizona. But when you stop exercising, you may not have enough blood circulating to your heart and brain. That can cause faintness. A cool-down allows your body to circulate blood out of the extremities and back to the vital parts that need it to function, says Dr. Wilmore.

"No pain, no gain" is a myth.

The safety tips we've mentioned have become the framework in recent years for a more relaxed approach to all forms of exercise. Gone are the days of "no pain, no gain"—an expression you may recall from school days. It's been replaced by an attitude among exercise experts of "all gain and no pain." They've seen enough of all kinds of exercise injuries to believe that none of us, recreational exercisers up to Olympic athletes, should be punishing our bodies to get the benefits of exercise.

And they've also discovered that even relatively low levels of physical activity, when performed on a regular basis, are associated with fewer cardiovascular problems in healthy people, as well as in people at high risk of strokes and heart attacks.

So don't think that exercise isn't for you, just because you're busy or you can't imagine yourself ever participating in a marathon or a swimming race. A humble daily walk is enough to put you head and shoulders above those who remain sedentary.

How to Stay Motivated

You've chosen the exercise you think you'll like best and that you'll stick to. You've eased into the new activity gradually. And you understand how important exercise can be to help you prevent a stroke. Then why, after several weeks of faithfully following your program, are you backsliding? Welcome to the hardest reality about exercise: Before it gets to be a habit—and even sometimes after—it can be incredibly hard to keep it up.

Because sticking with exercise is such a common problem—especially for beginners or people who haven't exercised for a while—exercise experts have spent a lot of time figuring out what keeps some people going while others seem to flag. Here's a quick rundown of their best tips. Choose the ones you think will work for you.

Eight tips for sticking with an exercise program.

Schedule exercise into your calendar. Make it like any other appointment or engagement. You might try sitting down at the beginning of each week and writing into your schedule the times that week when you plan to exercise. Almost every exercise expert mentions this tip as a way to keep your exercise program on track. "How many people would make a hair appointment and then miss it? You should take exercise at least that seriously," says Karma Kientzler, the executive fitness director at Canyon Ranch Spa in Tucson, Arizona.

Try scheduling exercise into the slowest part of your day, when you're most likely to keep to your commitment. If you have to miss a scheduled session, then immediately go to your calendar and write down a makeup date.

Seven Winter-Friendly Exercises

You pedaled all spring. You swam all summer. You walked all autumn. But now it's simply too cold to do a thing—or so you think. How are you going to exercise?

Walk the malls. Spend a couple of hours walking around malls. They're all over and, admit it, they can be a lot of fun. Some of them even open early for walkers or sponsor mall-walking clubs. Where else do you get the scenery and the controlled climate?

Find indoor attractions. Malls not your style? Well, if your town has a botanical garden, visit it. Walk from the tropical garden to the indoor desert and enjoy the scenery. Or how about visiting an aviary? Or the indoor cages at a zoo?

Join a health club. You know how lots of health clubs offer special trial memberships? Well, why don't you try one now? If you don't like it after a few months, then just don't sign up—by then, the weather will be nicer anyway.

And you might find out it's a lot of fun. You can swim, take dance classes, play with exotic machinery, relax in a sauna and make friends at many of these clubs. Or check out your local YMCA.

Start slowly and make it convenient. Although we've mentioned both of these tips through the chapter, they're worth mentioning again because they're so crucial to adhering to an exercise program. If you try to do too much too soon, you're likely to sideline yourself with an injury before you ever make it up to speed. And if you choose an exercise you think is good for you—but it's one you find boring or too difficult

Avoid exercise that's boring, hard or too time-consuming.

They usually have cheaper memberships and often offer classes.

Jump around at home. Stay in your home, turn down the heat, turn up the stereo and dance till the cows come home (or your family, whichever is first). Make a tape of your favorite "psych-up" tunes to keep you going. Pedal a stationary bike as you watch TV, listen to records or read the newspaper. Buy a mini-trampoline and bounce to your heart's content.

Hike. If you're a hiker, keep it up. The landscape during winter can offer some of the most beautiful scenery of the year. And the cold will be invigorating.

Ski. Or try some cross-country skiing lessons. It's the best aerobic workout you can get, but you can take it at your own pace—even if that means almost walking in the beginning, says Didi Yunginger, associate editor of Cross Country Skier magazine. Take a class, and you can be gliding through icy forests, parks and golf courses in no time.

Take advantage of the morning sun. And here's a motivator to make a morning walk more attractive: Sleep in your sweats. That way, leaving a warm bed to go out into the cold air won't be so much of a threat.

or too hard to find time for—you're asking for failure.

Set goals, keep track of your progress and reward yourself. Write down a goal for eack week or month. Make a contract with yourself to walk five days a week, for example. Then mark on your calendar or an exercise log when you complete every walk. When you reach your goal, reward yourself. Buy a new pair of walking shoes, or take yourself to a play or sporting event. Then make a new goal and work toward that. Studies have shown that people who do this are more likely to stick to exercising.

Reward your achievements.

If you've chosen walking as your exercise, you might be interested in the goal-and-reward system offered by the Prevention Magazine Walking Club, a part of Rodale Press. When you join, you get a daily log to record your progress toward goals, and when you reach those goals, the club offers rewards in the form of certificates and patches that recognize your achievements. There are awards for every level of accomplishment, so you don't have to be an experienced walker to participate.

There are also additional benefits to membership, including a quarterly newsletter on walking, an annual magazine and specially organized walking tours at various locations across the country. To join, write to the Prevention Walking Club, 33 East Minor Street, Emmaus, PA 18098, for details.

Work out with a group, or get a partner involved. Exercise research shows that nine out of ten people prefer to work out in a group instead of alone. So you might want to join an exercise class or invite your spouse or a friend to walk, run, bike or swim with you. When you're absorbed in conversation, time passes quickly and you avoid getting bored. A good partner or group probably won't let you get away with skipping your exercise session either!

Draft your friends.

Pretend you're walking (or running, biking, swimming) across the country. You can put up a map of the United States (or your own state if you prefer smaller goals) and chart your mileage as you exercise. You'd be amazed at how far you'll go. Think of the bragging you can indulge in: "I walked across four states this summer," you might say.

Use your imagination.

Psych yourself up. Professional athletes aren't the only ones who can profit from this motivational booster. About an hour before you plan to exercise, start to imagine yourself out there walking in the fresh air, swimming in the cool water or dancing your heart out. Remember how good and invigorated you feel afterward. Reflect on the physical and emotional benefits of exercising—remember you're helping to prevent a stroke! Then go for it.

Add variety to your program and keep it fun. If you find you're getting bored with your exercise routine, spice it up a little. Change your walking or running route. Attend a different dance class. Try water aerobics instead of swimming laps for a while. Or try a whole different type of exercise with all its new challenges. Remember, no one—including you—is going to keep up a program that isn't fun and something you look forward to doing.

Don't be afraid to change.

Be positive—don't quit just because you've stopped for a while. Everyone has times, whether because of family or work commitments, when exercise has to take a low priority. Don't get so discouraged that you wind up quitting altogether just because you've stopped exercising for a week or two. Pick up where you left off and ease back into the swing of things. Remember—nobody's perfect.

Nobody's perfect. Why should you be?

Chapter 6

Smoking and Heavy Drinking: Bad Habits Are Bad for Your Brain

The reports are in. New studies show alarming evidence that cigarettes and alcohol make you vulnerable to strokes. Smokers, for example, have a two to three times higher risk of stroke than nonsmokers. And it's a risk that keeps rising the more you smoke or drink. But those same studies that fingered smoking and drinking as stroke risk factors also discovered something exciting. People who managed to quit smoking or cut back on their drinking reduced their risk of stroke tremendously. One study showed, for example, that four to five years after they quit, ex-smokers had the *same* risk of stroke as those who had never smoked!

Quit smoking and you'll soon reduce your risk of stroke to that of a nonsmoker.

133

From that type of study, researchers theorize that the negative effects of cigarettes and alcohol on your cardiovascular system may be only temporary—that those effects stop when those habits stop.

Why are smoking and drinking so dangerous? One theory says that they can trigger the formation of stroke-causing blood clots. Clots develop when certain sticky cell fragments in the blood, called platelets, clump together and then adhere to the walls of your arteries. Smoking and heavy drinking make platelets even stickier than normal.

Smoking and drinking make the platelets in your blood stick together.

But this duo's dirty work doesn't end with clots. Smoking can constrict your arteries. Alcohol can make your heart beat irregularly. Both of these health insults can speed clots from the arteries of the heart to an artery supplying blood to the brain. And that, as you know, can lead to a stroke.

But don't think that clot prevention is the only reason to quit smoking and cut back on your drinking. Other studies show that cutting back on alcohol consumption helps some people lower their blood pressure. Since hypertension is the number one risk factor for stroke, that's a compelling reason to go easy on the bottle. And there are other health benefits. Studies of smokers who quit show that their risk of dying from heart disease diminishes with each year they stay off cigarettes. In addition, lighter drinking protects your liver, digestive tract and heart from the abuses of heavy alcohol consumption.

End smoker's cough and renew your sense of taste and smell.

And even when you set aside the health advantages, there are other day-to-day benefits to be gained. Ex-smokers report a renewed sense of taste and smell and an end to smoker's cough. They get fewer colds and flu bugs and they have a lot more energy.

So let's look at the latest research on how to rid yourself of a smoking habit and how to cut back on alcohol.

The Challenge of a Smoke-Free Life

When you quit smoking, there are two challenges you must face, says Nina Schneider, Ph.D., an associate research psychologist at the University of California at Los Angeles (UCLA) who has also developed smoking cessation programs for hospitals and health clinics. The first is the initial quitting stage, when you may feel the uncomfortable symptoms of withdrawal from nicotine—irritability, anxiety, depression, insomnia, gastrointestinal disorders—as well as the emotional and psychological loss of a long-time friend. But the second stage—maintaining a smoke-free life—is probably the bigger challenge.

"Everything in your life changes," says Dr. Schneider, who has done a great deal of research using nicotine gum to help smokers quit. "Because, if you're like most smokers, you probably use cigarettes both to cope with life and to reward yourself. Anger, stress, joy—all are accompanied by a cigarette. In fact, if you've been smoking since you were very young, you may *never* have developed other coping skills. Now, you need to learn new ways to reward yourself and to cope with anxiety and stress."

Everything changes when you quit.

And that process of relearning takes time. So don't worry if you've tried to quit smoking before and wound up going back to it. Dr. Schneider sees that as a positive sign. "I think a lot of people have to quit several times before they find out the best way to stay stopped," she says. "They learn when it's hardest to be without a cigarette and what caused them to relapse. That's the first step to self-enlightenment."

A lot of people have to quit several times before they find the best way to stay stopped.

If weight gain was your nemesis, for example, you'll know you need to be extra careful about the food you eat. Cigarette smokers have a higher metabolic rate—when you quit the rate falls and this contributes to weight gain. You need to remember that. Or if you had a hard time coping with stress and that caused you to start smoking again, then you know you'll need to develop different ways to deal with stress—learn a new way to relax or take up exercise to blow off steam. You get the idea.

"If you've quit several times, that's indeed an encouraging sign. If you did it before, you can do it again," says Jerome L. Schwartz, Dr.P.H. (doctor of public health), a smoking cessation expert who just wrote a review of smoking cessation methods for the National Cancer Institute. "Now, it's just a matter of doing it longer."

And you shouldn't feel alone or embarrassed that you tried to quit but couldn't hack it. Surveys show that the majority of smokers make at least one serious but unsuccessful attempt to stop smoking before they actually quit. So don't give up—you can do what 37 million other Americans have done already—get off cigarettes for good!

Successful "quitters" quit more than once.

How Do You Stop?

What's the best way to quit? The answer is different for each person, says Dr. Schneider. "Giving up cigarettes is like getting a divorce—you don't know whether you'll need help until you go through it." So she suggests quitting on your own first. "And please don't worry if you relapse. Remember, that's when you'll learn—you'll know what your traps are the next time around." Dr. Schwartz says that quitting on your own is worth trying, especially if you're a light smoker.

Stack the deck in your favor with tips from the pros.

But stack the deck in your favor. Groups like the American Lung Association, the American Cancer Society and others have devised self-help manuals that incorporate some of the best tips and ideas from smoking cessation experts on how to quit on your own. (See the box, "Organizations That Can Help You Quit," on page 142 for a list of these materials and where they can be obtained.) You'll learn strategies for quitting, ways to cope with smoking urges, how to prepare for situations when you know you'll want a cigarette, tips on keeping your weight down and more.

But if you're the kind of person who likes the motivation of working with a group or you feel you'd benefit from the hands-on help of a professional in the smoking cessation field, then you might want to opt instead for a smoking control program. All the effective tips and strategies will be explained and you'll have a chance to practice becoming a nonsmoker with a very sympathetic group.

Get the hands-on help of a professional—or the sympathetic support of a group.

You can find smoking control programs in many locations these days. Local cancer, lung and heart associations sponsor them, as do hospitals, colleges, medical centers, community agencies and exercise clubs. (See the box, "Organizations That Can Help You Quit," on page 142 for some sources.) There are also commercial programs, many of which are found in the yellow pages of your phone book.

If you're lucky, your employers may offer a smoking control program, perhaps in conjunction with a new policy that restricts smoking in the workplace. And if they don't, why don't you suggest it?

Get your workplace involved.

Many companies are finding it makes sense to help employees quit because smokers cost them more money in insurance claims, absenteeism, even routine office cleaning. No more ashtrays to dump and wash, right? And worksite programs may ultimately be the most effective. They're easy to get to, Dr. Schneider points out, and your co-workers are around to give you moral support. Moreover, if your company restricts smoking, you won't be as tempted to smoke. "I think worksite smoking restrictions will guarantee more success to everyone who quits," says Dr. Schneider.

How Can You Handle Withdrawal?

Even armed with all the education and moral support in the world, you may still feel unable to cope with the withdrawal symptoms many people suffer when they give up smoking. You're not alone. "We're just now beginning to realize how addictive a substance nicotine really is," says chest physician David P. Sachs, M.D., director of the Smoking Cessation Research Institute at the Palo Alto Center for Pulmonary Disease Prevention. "Ounce for ounce nicotine has a stronger addictive effect on the body than any drug being sold illegally on the street today."

Because of this new awareness, says Dr. Schneider, "people are coming to realize that what they're caught in is a drug dependency situation. They're *not* weak-willed."

But if you're having trouble dealing with withdrawal symptoms, you may want to ask your doctor to write you a prescription for nicotine gum. The gum keeps just enough nicotine in your system to take the edge off withdrawal. And Dr. Schneider points out that even though you're still taking in nicotine while you chew, it's a much lower dose. Also, you've eliminated the other damaging constituents of smoke and you've given yourself time to adjust to life as a nonsmoker—without having to deal with physical withdrawal. Moreover, the gum also seems to prevent much of the weight gain frequently associated with withdrawal.

Studies have shown that nicotine gum can nearly *double* your chances of being able to quit and stay smoke-free when its use is combined with behavioral training—learning new, no-cigarette ways to cope with stress, learning what to do when you have the urge to smoke.

How do you use nicotine gum effectively? It's extremely important to follow your doctor's in-

Nicotine is more addictive than street drugs.

Nicotine gum may ease your transition into a smoke-free life.

structions because you must use the gum correctly to get its benefits. Among the things he will probably advise: You should chew the gum slowly whenever you feel the need to smoke and keep chewing each piece for 20 to 30 minutes—that's how long it takes to release most of the nicotine. Make sure you chew enough gum to provide steady relief of withdrawal symptoms, advises Dr. Schneider. Use a minimum of 8 to 15 pieces a day for the first month but never more than 30 a day for the entire time you're on the program. And don't be in too much of a hurry to wean yourself from the gum, says Dr. Schneider. Many people stop too soon and then go back to smoking. Give yourself several months of gradually reducing the amount you use.

Chew each piece of gum for 20 to 30 minutes.

And don't let the gum's side effects discourage you. Chewing slowly can help you avoid the hiccups, nausea, flatulence and mouth and gum soreness that occasionally occur.

Chew slowly to avoid the gum's side effects.

Whether you experience side effects or not, nicotine gum isn't recommended for ulcer patients, people with very serious heart conditions, those with temporomandibular joint disorders and pregnant or nursing women. Your doctor can help you decide if the gum is for you.

Using Your Mind

What about hypnosis to help you stop smoking? California's Dr. Schwartz surveyed telephone book yellow pages across the country for his review of smoking cessation methods and found that hypnosis was the most frequently advertised method to quit smoking. But it's hard to evaluate the effectiveness of hypnosis since studies haven't always followed people long enough to see if they stay off cigarettes. Although the evidence suggests that hypnosis may be only modestly effective

Hypnosis is more successful when combined with other techniques.

when used alone, it's more successful when coupled with other smoking cessation techniques.

How do hypnotists try to help smokers quit? There are many ways, reports Dr. Schwartz. While you're hypnotized, you could be told to think of something disgusting every time you want to smoke. Or you could simply learn to automatically relax yourself every time you feel the urge to smoke. Then, when you come out of hypnosis, hopefully those suggestions would stay with you.

Make yourself sick of smoking.

Another method that has met with some success is a doctor-implemented program called aversive smoking. Under supervision from a professional, you smoke so rapidly that smoking ceases to be pleasurable. In fact, it makes you sick. So sick you never want to smoke again.

This technique can put quite a strain on your heart and lungs, however, so you have to be carefully screened before doing it. As with other stop-smoking techniques, aversive smoking works best when it's combined with behavioral instructions that teach you how to function without a cigarette in your hand, observes Dr. Schwartz.

Staying a Quitter

So far, we've focused on how to quit smoking—especially those first crucial weeks and months after you stop. But be careful—you're not out of the woods yet. "Once the smoker abstains, a myriad of forces act upon the individual, influencing him to return to smoking," says Dr. Schwartz. "These forces include environmental, social and internal pressures from advertisements, friends and everyday stress. When the smoker breaks his habit, he still has to deal with his possibly intense urges to smoke. This is why maintenance is so important. And difficult."

Keep your guard up.

What he means is that even after your withdrawal symptoms go away—even after you've gone three or four or even six months without smoking—you still need to be on guard. That's

why experts who study smoking cessation programs are now insisting that to be considered
really valid, studies of stop-smoking programs and
techniques should follow ex-smokers for at least
six months to a year to see which people are really
able to stay smoke-free.

Why do people light up after they've quit?
Common reasons include the inability to deal with
anger, anxiety and depression, and missing cigarettes at specific times, such as at meals or when
sipping a cocktail.

That's why smoking control programs are de-
voting more and more time to helping ex-smokers
stay off cigarettes for good. The two most important ingredients for success, agree Drs. Schneider
and Schwartz, are learning how to handle the urge
to smoke and getting support from family, friends,
co-workers and others to stay off cigarettes.

"Everything you do will feel phony at first,"
says Dr. Schneider. "Because you're substituting
for that familiar cigarette. But if you don't plan
coping strategies and you're caught off guard
when you feel really stressed or worried about
something, you'll probably wind up smoking." So
here are some widely used techniques to help you
deal with your urges to smoke.

Plan what you'll do when the urge hits.

List your reasons for quitting. These might
include lowering your risk of stroke, heart attack
and cancer. Or because close family members
really want you to do it. Or to save money. Or to
regain your sense of taste and smell. Add as many
reasons as possible and then keep the list handy.
When you feel the urge to smoke, you can look at
it as a reminder and a motivator.

**Keep a record of when you feel the urge to
smoke.** You'll gain real insight into what triggers
your craving for a cigarette.

Work out your coping strategies. If you usually smoke after meals, get up from the table and
take a walk instead. If work stress makes you want
a cigarette, learn to take a deep breath and let your
craving flow out of your body along with the air

Take a deep breath and let your craving flow out of your body as you exhale.

Organizations that Can Help You Quit

Looking for help and support materials to quit smoking? There are several excellent resources.

The National Cancer Institute. The institute's toll-free Cancer Information Service number (1-800-4-CANCER) can help you locate the institute office nearest you. Trained personnel can give you the information you need to quit. Or write to the Office of Cancer Communications, National Cancer Institute, National Institutes of Health, Building 31, Room 10A24, Bethesda, MD 20892.

American Cancer Society (ACS). This voluntary organization has a variety of materials to help you quit, including a printed *7-Day Plan to Help You Stop Smoking Cigarettes* and local smoking cessation group programs called FreshStart. For information on the FreshStart program nearest you or to obtain written self-help materials, contact the local chapter of the ACS listed in your phone book.

American Lung Association (ALA). The ALA is also a voluntary organization with a tremendous interest in helping people to stop smoking. It offers several written guides to help you stop smoking including *Freedom from Smoking*

you exhale. And try to avoid places where a lot of smoking goes on, since seeing others smoking is usually a powerful trigger.

These are just a few examples of how to cope with your smoking triggers. Spend some time now looking over your record of cigarette craving and think of additional ways to deal with those moments. Here are a few suggestions.

- Exercise. It gives you something to do instead of smoking. It's good for you and

in 20 Days, a comprehensive manual that gives detailed instructions for quitting in a gradual fashion.

The ALA's newest quit-smoking manual is called *Freedom from Smoking for You and Your Family.* This guidebook contains somewhat easier instructions and is more concisely written than the manual. It also seems to have a few words of wisdom for people who have tried everything. The ALA also offers a home video called *In Control,* which was developed in consultation with Nina Schneider, Ph.D., the UCLA smoking cessation specialist mentioned in this chapter.

Finally, the organization also offers stop-smoking groups where you meet with others who want to quit. For information on all of the ALA's stop-smoking programs, look in your phone book for the American Lung Association chapter closest to you.

Office on Smoking and Health (OSH). The Office on Smoking and Health is a federal department that distributes free pamphlets on smoking-related topics, including how to deal with smoking relapses after you quit, helping a friend or family member quit smoking and the effects of parental smoking on teenagers. Write to Office on Smoking and Health, Centers for Disease Control, 1-10 Park Building, 2600 Fishers Lane, Rockville, MD 20857. The information is free.

you'll feel healthier, too. It substitutes a good habit for a bad habit and it fits right into your stroke-prevention program. (See chapter 5 for how to get started.)

- Decide how you'll deal with overeating. If you're changing your eating habits along the lines of the program we suggested in chapter 4, weight gain shouldn't be a problem. But it bears repeating that if you use food to satisfy your oral craving for a ciga-

Eat popcorn or fruit.

rette, let it be with popcorn, fruit and other low-calorie nibbles—not candy and potato chips.

- Learn a relaxation technique. Since stress is one of the most common reasons people reach for a cigarette, it pays to develop new ways of dealing with it. Here's a simple relaxation technique suggested by the American Lung Association: Think about something that makes you feel good. Relax your shoulders, close your mouth and inhale as slowly and deeply as you can. Hold your breath as you count to four, then exhale slowly. Repeat five times.

- Reward yourself. Be good to yourself. Indulge in activities you love. Buy yourself something you've been wanting. See friends. These are just a few suggestions—use your imagination to think of things you really want.

Use your imagination to think up a just reward.

Along with developing ways to cope with not smoking, you should also enlist the help of those around you. This kind of social support can be crucial to your success. Many experts suggest that you choose a buddy—someone you can call when you're feeling an overwhelming urge to smoke. Your buddy can cheer you on, praise your success and help keep you motivated. In fact, you may want to have several "buddies"—located in all the places you'll be.

Your family can help at home. Friends can help at parties. Co-workers can help on the job. At any rate, tell them all that you've quit smoking. And ask them not to offer you a cigarette or give you one if you ask for it.

You can do it with a little help from friends.

What about people who aren't supportive? Some people may not even realize that they're hampering your efforts. Don't despair, for instance, if you meet people who tell you they're still craving a cigarette ten years after they quit.

"It's really unfair of people to say that, especially to someone who is still in the throes of quitting," says Dr. Schneider. Those cravings are occasional and will pass in a moment, and will subside as the days and months go by.

But what if you slip and find yourself looking at the burnt end of a cigarette? Shrug your shoulders and get on with your life. So you've had a small setback—that doesn't make you a bad person. Start right back where you left off and remember how far you've already come.

Ignore the nicotine saboteur.

Alcohol and Stroke

If you're a smoker, one of the most common triggers that can cause you to want a cigarette is a drink. So if you're trying to quit, cutting back on your drinking can help. But that's not the only reason to curb your alcohol intake. In terms of stroke, one study found that there was a fourfold increased risk of stroke among people who drank 30 drinks or more a week.

Alcohol can quadruple your risk of stroke.

And alcohol can harm your brain in other ways, especially by impairing your memory and other cognitive functions, according to the U.S. Department of Health and Human Services' Sixth Special Report to the U.S. Congress on Alcohol and Health. There's the safety factor, too. Alcohol is a major factor in traffic accidents, house fires and falls.

And then there's the happiness angle. Although alcohol in small quantities can make you feel like a social butterfly, in large doses it can make you feel more like an inept elephant. And excessive alcohol can lead to major bouts of depression. Moreover, it can make you fat. Did you know that a single shot (1¼ ounces) of 80-proof liquor packs a hefty 120 calories?

Heavy drinking can make you feel like an inept elephant.

There's also the monetary incentive. Drinking two fifths a week can amount to over $800 a year.

That amount of drinking paid for by the glass in bars and restaurants can cost over $3,200 a year!

What are we talking about when we say "cut back"? For one thing, it means not drinking every day. Or not drinking too much at any one sitting.

Habitual drinkers may not realize exactly how much it takes to mellow them out.

Why? Studies have shown that both habitual daily consumption or binge drinking seem to be related to deaths from stroke and coronary heart disease. In addition, daily drinkers can unknowingly become so tolerant of alcohol that they must increase their intake to achieve the same mellow feelings they used to experience after a few sips.

Along with not drinking every day, try not to drink for more than an hour at any one sitting. If you drink much longer than that, you'll probably consume an unhealthful amount. And the mild pleasantness or "high" that you feel will fade.

Another good rule of thumb is to drink only one drink per hour, or two to three drinks over three hours, advises Richard J. Bast, senior technical advisor for the National Clearinghouse for Alcohol and Drug Information. That will give your body enough time to metabolize each drink. Better still, choose an hour when you'll drink and then switch to nonalcoholic beverages for the rest of the time.

Don't drink when you're feeling bad.

And try to limit your drinking only to times when you feel it will enhance your already-good feelings. Don't drink when you're already feeling bad, in the hopes of making things better. Using alcohol as a "cure" is the first step to making drinking a disease.

Besides these health-enhancing ways to keep your alcohol consumption under control, there are other ways to avoid drinking too much, especially at events when alcohol tends to take center stage. Many people wind up drinking more than they really want on such occasions, so here are a few common situations and how to get around them.

The ubiquitous cocktail hour. Now here's an event designed to sabotage anyone's liquor control effort. "Hour" is a misnomer—most of them last nearly two, if not longer. Leave early, if you can, and schedule a meeting or other appointment to use as your excuse. Or, arrive late. You could also alternate between booze and water while you're there. You'll always have something in your hand to sip, but you'll get only half the liquor.

Another alternative is to dilute your drinks. Start out with a regular drink, but add water or club soda when it's half empty. Every time your glass is half empty again, dilute it once more.

Add club soda every time your drink's half empty.

And make sure you go to the bar to order your drinks, rather than from a server. It takes more effort to go to the bar and you may be so engrossed in conversation you'll forget to do it.

Finally, try sipping your drink slowly. A warm martini, flat gin and tonic or watery Bloody Mary isn't very appealing. So the longer your drink lasts, the less you'll feel like finishing it.

When you dine out. Don't feel pressured to have a before-meal cocktail. Save your palate for a glass of really fine wine and then savor it slowly with your food. This is definitely an example of drinking less and enjoying it more. If you're dining with people who you know will insist you drink, arrive earlier than they do and order a well-disguised nonalcoholic drink (like a Bloody Mary without the vodka) to have in hand. If you're meeting someone for lunch and you'd rather not have a drink, tell them you have an important meeting or deal to complete that afternoon. Most people will be impressed with your professionalism.

You can avoid social drinking with a little forethought.

At business functions. Although business entertaining traditionally used to mean a lot of drinking, that's changed in recent years. And it pays to come up with ways to entertain clients that don't revolve around liquor. If they're not doing it—you won't have to either. Although many people appreciate a drink to loosen up at business functions, there are others ways to achieve this end. Take clients for a walk around your company, especially if you have beautiful grounds or

Relax your clients with walks, not booze.

Special Help for Problem Drinkers

Alcohol-control tips, such as those discussed in this chapter, are often enough to keep people imbibing within reasonable limits. But some of us may be drinking way beyond those limits now, and cutting back doesn't seem to work. How do you know if you're that kind of person?

Richard J. Bast, senior technical advisor for the National Clearinghouse for Alcohol and Drug Information, says problem drinkers are, first and foremost, people who drink despite possible dangers to their health and welfare. Ask yourself these other questions—yes answers are signs that you may have a serious drinking problem.

- Are you getting into drinking-related trouble with family and friends, at work and/or with the police?
- Do you experience withdrawal symptoms, such as sweating, shaking and trembling?
- Do you have to drink until you're drunk or unconscious?
- Do you binge? Do you stay sober for a few weeks and then binge again?
- Are you unable to stop drinking despite promises to yourself and others to do so?

Recognize yourself? If you do—take heart, and take action. There are lots of people and orga-

an unusual facility. If you're in a city, suggest a walk through an art gallery, museum or park. All these outings give you a lot to comment on, relaxing your clients and readying them for the business discussion ahead.

You can also have lunch sent in when you're involved in an important meeting. And it doesn't

nizations around that can help you get sober for good. You can begin to get help by consulting with your family doctor or a member of the clergy. If you have an employee assistance program at work, it can also put you in touch with someone who can help you, in strictest confidence. Here are some other good resources for help and information.

Alcoholics Anonymous. Through this voluntary fellowship, alcoholics help themselves and each other get sober and stay sober. Just look in your phone book for the chapter nearest you, or contact the world services office of Alcoholics Anonymous, P.O. Box 459, Grand Central Station, Park Avenue, New York, NY 10163.

National Council on Alcoholism. This organization distributes literature and can refer you to treatment sources in your area. Check your telephone book for a local number or write to National Council on Alcoholism, 12 West Twenty-first Street, Suite 700, New York, NY 10010.

National Clearinghouse for Alcohol and Drug Information. This government-funded organization can also provide you with information and resources. Write the National Clearinghouse for Alcohol and Drug Information, P.O. Box 2345, Rockville, MD 20852.

have to be deli sandwiches either. Many caterers can deliver elegant lunches for such occasions and people rarely expect liquor at them. But if you're not going to have liquor at a business event, be sure to provide sophisticated and exciting nonalcoholic beverages. Have lots of fresh fruit garnishes, mineral waters, mint leaves and fruit juices available.

You can probably negotiate better over mineral water than alcohol.

You could also try nonalcoholic beers and wines, which are growing in popularity.

Finally, consider meeting at times when liquor isn't expected—over breakfast or at a late afternoon tea where food and hot drinks are served. Or, if you expect to do more entertaining than negotiating, take your guests to nonfood events like a horse show, golf tournament, the theater or a concert. It'll be much easier than going to the typical liquor-laden dinner.

Renew your energy.

Alcohol, like smoking, is a habit you can learn to control—before it controls you. If you're a heavy drinker, give moderate drinking a try. You'll find your energy renewed and your spirits uplifted. And best of all, you'll reduce your risk of having a stroke.

Chapter 7

A Guide to Stroke-Prevention Drugs

The best way to prevent a stroke is self-care—the diet, exercise and lifestyle changes we've recommended in this book. But if you've suffered a transient ischemic attack, or TIA (those brief, strokelike attacks we described in chapter 3), it may be time for *medical* care. Your doctor may want to prescribe a drug that can keep you from suffering a full-blown stroke. That's because a stroke is now a very real possibility: People who've had TIAs are about *ten* times more likely to have a stroke than people who haven't had TIAs.

The warning signs of a TIA, you may recall, are any one or a combination of these symptoms: You feel weak or numb in your face or any part of one or more limbs; you lose the ability to speak clearly and/or have trouble understanding the speech of others; you experience dimness or loss of vision; you feel dizzy or unsteady or you suddenly fall.

Doctors sometimes give stroke-prevention medicine to people who've had those kinds of

People who've had TIAs are ten times more likely to have strokes.

151

symptoms and sometimes even to those who've had tests that document the presence of a clogged neck artery—a sign they might have a TIA or stroke in the future.

Another group that may be treated is people with certain heart conditions—atrial fibrillation, for example—that predispose them to blood clots forming in the heart. Doctors try to prevent those heart clots from traveling to the brain, where they could become lodged in an artery and cause what's called an embolic stroke.

Drugs can prevent strokes by "thinning" your blood.

Regardless of the reason, the two kinds of drugs doctors use most in treating people at risk for stroke are anti-platelet-aggregating drugs (aspirin is the most effective) and anticoagulant drugs such as coumarin. Both work to "thin" the blood and prevent the dangerous clots that cause so many strokes.

But even before doctors started using blood thinners, they'd be very likely to double-check your blood pressure, even if it had been normal at your last medical checkup. If they found it was elevated, they would very carefully give you medicines to reduce it to normal, since high blood pressure increases your risk of stroke so much, says Mark L. Dyken, Jr., M.D., chairman of the Department of Neurology at Indiana University and past chairman of the Stroke Council of the American Heart Association.

Let's look more closely at each drug, starting with aspirin.

Aspirin: Policing Your Platelets

Cell-sized lifesavers.

Platelets, disk-shaped cell fragments in your blood, can save your life if you're involved in an accident. That's because they immediately go to the site where you're bleeding and, by sticking together, cause your blood to clot. The bleeding stops. But in arteries damaged by atherosclerosis and high blood pressure, those same lifesavers can be life-threatening. They can become an unruly crowd, threatening to riot as too many of them jam together around damaged spots in your arteries. As the pileup increases, so does your risk of a dangerous clot forming at the site—a clot that can cut off the blood supply to your brain and cause a stroke.

When platelets clump together to cause clotting, that process is called "platelet aggregation." And that's where aspirin comes in. Like a police officer called to break up that unruly crowd, aspirin acts to keep the platelets from sticking together.

Doctors discovered aspirin's effect on dangerous blood clots when they saw that people who took aspirin seemed to have fewer heart attacks than average. (Heart attacks can be caused by blood clots in the arteries.) So scientists began to study whether the anticlotting properties of aspirin could stop heart attacks and strokes in people at high risk. In 1985, after reviewing seven studies, federal health officials announced that taking one aspirin (about 325 mg) a day could help some heart attack victims reduce the likelihood of a second attack.

An aspirin a day can keep a heart attack at bay.

Then in 1988, another study found that even among healthy male physicians who had not suffered heart attacks, just one aspirin every other day made it much less likely that they would fall prey to a heart attack than another similar group which did not take aspirin.

And now there's overwhelming evidence that you can also reduce your chances of suffering a stroke by 25 to 30 percent if you take aspirin after a TIA, according to James C. Grotta, M.D., a neurologist at the University of Texas Medical School in Houston, who recently reviewed medical and surgical therapies for stroke-related disease in the *New England Journal of Medicine*.

Aspirin can reduce your risk of stroke 25 to 30 percent after a TIA.

In one study on stroke and aspirin, researchers investigated aspirin's effect on large groups of people who'd had TIAs. They gave some people aspirin and some a drug look-alike (placebo). A follow-up check several years later revealed that those taking aspirin had many fewer strokes. Aspirin was particularly effective against the kind of stroke that results from atherosclerosis of the arteries that supply blood to the brain, according to Robert Hart, M.D., a neurologist at the University of Texas Health Science Center, San Antonio.

It may work best on its own.

Researchers also found that two other antiplatelet-aggregation agents, the drugs dipyridamole and sulfinpyrazone, did nothing to enhance the effect of aspirin on blood clotting. Doctors at one time thought these other drugs would help prevent strokes. (However, dipyridamole and other drugs are often prescribed for the stroke-prone by doctors who are treating these same people for heart disease. Since the two problems so often occur simultaneously, check with your doctor to be sure.)

Along the way, researchers discovered something paradoxical about aspirin. Aspirin actually has both a positive and a negative effect. The good news is that it blocks an enzyme in platelets that produces the biochemical thromboxane, which makes platelets clump together and arteries constrict—the dangerous scenario that causes so many strokes and heart attacks. But the bad news is that the same aspirin-sensitive enzyme is also present in the walls of the arteries. There, it's used to produce a biochemical called prostacyclin, which *unclumps* platelets and *dilates* arteries.

Platelets won't stick or clump together.

Fortunately, platelets appear to be more sensitive to aspirin than are artery walls. So the challenge has been to find the correct dosage of aspirin that will inhibit the chemical agent that makes platelets stick together, while leaving undisturbed the other chemical substance which unclumps platelets.

Scientists knew, based on their work in the lab, that lower doses of aspirin would be better for doing this. But they also needed to see if lower doses would still prevent strokes in large numbers of high-risk people. And that's exactly what a project called the UK/TIA study tried to find out.

More than 60 neurologists in England and Scotland agreed to cooperate in the study of almost 2,500 of their patients who had experienced TIAs or mild strokes. They gave some patients a high dosage of aspirin—1,200 mg, or close to four aspirin tablets a day. This was similar to the doses given in other large aspirin studies that showed aspirin to be effective in preventing strokes. Other patients got only 300 mg of aspirin, closer to one tablet a day. A third group of patients got a nontherapeutic placebo that merely looked like aspirin.

What's the correct dose?

"Although in their report they noted no difference in beneficial effect between low-dose and high-dose aspirin, they stated, 'We could not definitely exclude a real difference between the two active treatment arms . . . ' If this lack of difference could be supported by further studies, then many doctors would routinely place their patients on lower-dose aspirin," says Dr. Dyken.

Why are doctors excited by this? If it could be confirmed that lower doses of aspirin are as effective, says Dr. Dyken, it also would mean fewer side effects for people taking aspirin. If you have stomach problems like ulcers, for example, you may not be able to tolerate a high dose of aspirin despite the fact that it could help you prevent a stroke. But lower doses mean less stomach irritation.

A lower dose means more people can use it to prevent strokes.

What's the bottom line on when and how much aspirin to take if you're at risk for a stroke? Although all the experts we interviewed for this chapter cautioned that those questions are best answered by a doctor who has evaluated your particular case, a few general statements can be made.

If you've had a TIA, you may be placed on an aspirin regimen of anywhere from one to four tablets a day. (As we said, if the final results of the UK/TIA trial are convincing, your doctor may opt for a lower dosage.) Dr. Dyken says he still starts

Some doctors feel people who've had TIAs should take four aspirin a day.

all his TIA patients on four aspirin (1,300 mg) a day, unless they can't tolerate it. In that case, he cuts back to one (325 mg) a day. If they still have problems, he opts for one baby aspirin a day (80 mg), which studies have shown is still effective in keeping platelets from clumping together.

Aspirin and Arteries that Talk

There's help for noisy arteries.

What if you haven't had a TIA, but a doctor listens to your carotid arteries with a stethoscope and hears an abnormal sound called a bruit in one of them? Well, a bruit is a sign that fatty deposits are building up within that artery due to atherosclerosis. And, since it does indicate you're more likely to have a stroke than someone with a quieter artery, many doctors prescribe aspirin for patients who have bruits. But there's no study showing that *any* particular medicine—or surgery for that matter—is effective or ineffective in preventing strokes in these people," says Harold P. Adams, Jr., M.D., professor of neurology and director of the Division of Cerebrovascular Diseases, University of Iowa, Iowa City.

"The rationale many doctors use is that, since aspirin is a fairly benign medicine and it's effective on people who have already had TIAs, why not give it a try?"

Until it's established, you may want to discuss with your doctor the option of taking one aspirin a day if you have a bruit. That's the dose many authorities recommend, according to Anthony J. Furlan, M.D., director of the Cleveland Clinic's Cerebrovascular Program.

Doctors are taking aspirin themselves.

If you have no bruit but you do have high blood pressure, signs of heart disease or other risk factors for stroke, a doctor may still suggest that you take aspirin. But, again, there's no evidence either in cases like these that aspirin will definitely help prevent a stroke. And some medical authorities still caution against the widespread use of aspirin, since it does have side effects. Nevertheless, says Dr. Adams, many doctors themselves are taking aspirin as a preventive measure against stroke and heart attack.

Anticoagulants: Use with Caution

Like aspirin, anticoagulant medications also work to prevent clotting, but by different methods than anti-platelet aggregation. Anticoagulants are used much more cautiously than aspirin, however, because they're considerably more powerful and can actually cause strokes in some people.

Anticoagulants are more powerful than aspirin.

Anticoagulants, explains Dr. Dyken, can make it so difficult for your blood to clot that it doesn't even do it when it really needs to. And anticoagulants can often instigate bleeding in the brain, which can trigger the most serious and often fatal kind of stroke: the cerebral hemorrhage.

The risk of major bleeding episodes ranged from 2 to 22 percent in patients who had experienced TIAs or minor strokes and used anticoagulants for long periods of time, a recent review of studies found. And, even more alarming, 2 to 9 percent of these patients died. Patients with high blood pressure were especially vulnerable, since the effects of this disease make the brain more prone to bleeding.

People with high blood pressure seem more susceptible to the side effects of anticoagulants.

The authors of that review, which was published in the journal *Stroke*, also pointed out that patients with TIAs and minor strokes have a stroke and death risk of between 5 and 10 percent. Yet similar patients who are on anticoagulants wind up having just about the same risk because of bleeding problems. The authors' conclusion: "The present evidence does not support the use of long-term anticoagulant therapy in patients with transient cerebral ischemia [TIA] or minor strokes."

The risks of long-term anticoagulants may outweigh their advantages.

But, according to the stroke experts we consulted, there are some exceptions. The biggest one, says Dr. Dyken, is if doctors suspect that you had a

TIA because a clot broke loose from your heart, traveled to an artery supplying your brain, got stuck and triggered the TIA. There's a 50 percent chance that this kind of episode will happen again in the following year. And doctors believe you can prevent it by taking anticoagulants.

Another reason doctors may want to put you on a long-term regimen of anticoagulant drugs, adds Dr. Adams, is if you keep having TIAs even after you're put on aspirin therapy. Or if after you have a TIA, doctors discover that your carotid arteries are severely blocked because of atherosclerosis and you either don't want to or can't (because of poor health) have surgery to clean those arteries. (See chapter 8.) Then, concludes Dr. Adams, the risk of going on to have a stroke may be greater than the risk of anticoagulant drugs.

The anticoagulant drug that doctors frequently use under these circumstances is coumarin, sold under the trade names Panwarfin, Coumadin and Dicumarol. (See the table, "Drugs That Prevent Strokes," on page 160 for more information.)

Although doctors frown on prescibing anticoagulants for extended use, there are many doctors who give anticoagulants such as heparin on a short-term basis after a TIA. Anticoagulants are usually not quite as risky when used this way, and the rationale is this: Why not prescribe them right after a TIA when the risk of stroke is highest, then stop prescribing them as the risk for stroke goes down?

But there's not much in the way of firm evidence to support this practice, says Dr. Adams, and many doctors feel that it doesn't reduce the risk of stroke any more than doses of aspirin.

There are a few circumstances, however, when even if you *haven't* experienced a TIA, doctors might consider giving you anticoagulants to prevent a stroke. People with certain heart conditions that predispose them to produce clots are often placed on anticoagulants to prevent those

If aspirin doesn't work, anticoagulants may be an alternative.

People with heart disease may be put on anticoagulants to prevent strokes.

clots from traveling to the brain and causing a stroke. So are those with rheumatic and other heart valve diseases, and people who've had heart attacks, especially the type of heart damage which indicates that clots are probably going to develop afterward.

(continued on page 167)

A Drug Better than Aspirin?

Although aspirin is still considered the safest and most effective drug for keeping platelets from sticking together and causing the blood clots that lead to strokes, stroke prevention experts have continued to look for other drugs that might do the job even better. And the drug ticlopidine, doctors are hoping, may be the answer.

While aspirin blocks production of thromboxane, a biochemical that makes platelets stick together, it also blocks another biochemical called prostacyclin, which *unclumps* platelets. But what if researchers could develop another drug which didn't affect prostacyclin at all?

Enter ticlopidine. This new drug, which is still being tested, keeps platelets from sticking together by an altogether different process than aspirin—one that doesn't involve the production of prostacyclin, says James C. Grotta, M.D., a neurologist at the University of Texas Medical School, Houston.

A large study of patients who've had transient ischemic attacks—those strokelike attacks that put you at high risk for a real stroke—is under way, pitting ticlopidine against aspirin to see how effective the new drug is in preventing strokes. If ticlopidine proves its worth, the U.S. Food and Drug Administration will then begin evaluating it to compare its effectiveness to possible risk. According to recent reports, ticlopidine may have some serious side effects, so it may be a few years before doctors know for sure if they can use this drug. But for now, it's the newest hope for stroke prevention in the drug world.

Drugs That Prevent Strokes

Generic Name/ Brand Name	How Given	Benefits and Uses	Side Effects	Interactions/ Precautions
Aspirin (acetylsalicylic acid)	Available over-the-counter; prescribed by doctors for stroke prevention in doses up to 4 regular aspirin (325 mg each) a day. See your doctor for the dosage right for you.	Aspirin is an *anti-platelet aggregating agent*, which means it prevents stroke by keeping blood substances called platelets from sticking together and forming dangerous clots. (Strokes are mainly caused by clots which block the blood supply to the brain.)	Get emergency help immediately if these side effects occur: • any loss of hearing • bloody urine • confusion • severe or continuing drowsiness, nervousness, dizziness, nausea, vomiting or diarrhea • hallucinations • seizures • troubled breathing • unexplained fever • vision problems • unusual sweating, breathing or thirst • unusual or uncontrollable flapping movements of the hands	Before taking aspirin, check with your doctor if you are: • allergic to any medicines • on a special diet or allergic to any substance • pregnant or nursing • suffering from other medical problems (like heart disease, high blood pressure, kidney disease, stomach ulcer or other stomach problems, gout or any other disease) • taking other medicines, including over-the-counter drugs, or vitamins Here's how to properly use aspirin:

Check with your doctor if these side effects occur:

- nausea, vomiting or stomach pain
- bloody or black, tarry stools
- severe or continuing headaches or ringing/buzzing in the ears
- skin rashes, hives, itching
- unusual tiredness or weakness
- vomiting blood or material that looks like coffee grounds

- Take it after meals or with food to lessen stomach irritation.
- Take tablets with 8 oz. water.
- Don't use aspirin with a strong, vinegarlike odor. This means the medicine is breaking down.

Other precautions:

- Aspirin contains substances called salicylates, which are contained in many other drugs, too. So check labels on all prescription and over-the-counter drugs. If any contain salicylates, check with your doctor or pharmacist to ensure that you aren't taking too much.
- Check with your doctor before taking aspirin in the 5-day period before any surgery, since aspirin can cause bleeding problems.

(continued)

Drugs That Prevent Strokes—Continued

Generic Name/Brand Name	How Given	Benefits and Uses	Side Effects	Interactions/Precautions

Coumarin (also called warfarin) Common brand names: Panwarfin Coumadin Dicumarol	Available by prescription only, usually in tablet form. The prescribed amount is determined by your blood clotting time.	Coumarin-type drugs are *anticoagulants*, which prevent stroke by reducing the tendency of your blood to clot. This reduces the chance of dangerous clots forming in your arteries and blocking off the blood supply to your brain. Anticoagulants keep blood from clotting by helping keep platelets apart—but by a different means than aspirin.	The most serious side effect of anticoagulants is that by reducing the tendency of your blood to clot, they can actually cause you to bleed too easily. If that happens in your brain, a stroke could occur. Your doctor will regularly test your blood to be sure it's still clotting safely, but you should contact him immediately if these side effects occur:
			
			• bleeding from gums when brushing teeth
			• unexplained bruising or purplish areas on skin
			• unexplained nosebleeds
			• unusually heavy bleeding or oozing from cuts or wounds
			• unusually heavy or unexpected menstrual bleeding
				Before taking coumarin anticoagulants, make sure your doctor knows if you are:
				
				• allergic to anticoagulant medications
				• on a special diet or allergic to any substance
				• pregnant or nursing
				• suffering from any medical problems
				• taking any medicines, including over-the-counter drugs, or vitamins
				• recovering from or have recently had any of the following:
				  —childbirth
				  —falls or blows to the body or head
				  —fever lasting more than a few days
				  —heavy or unusual menstrual bleeding

- abdominal or stomach pain or swelling
- back pain or backaches
- bloody urine
- bloody or black, tarry stools
- constipation
- coughing up blood
- dizziness
- headache (severe or continuing)
- joint pain, stiffness or swelling
- vomiting blood or material that looks like coffee grounds

Also check with your doctor immediately if these infrequent or rare side effects occur:

- blue or purple toes, or pain in toes
- cloudy or dark urine
- difficult or painful urination
- sores, ulcers or white spots in mouth or throat
- sore throat and fever or chills
- sudden decrease in amount of urine

—insertion of an intrauterine device (IUD)

—medical or dental surgery

—severe or continuing diarrhea

—spinal anesthesia

—x-ray (radiation) treatment

Here's how to properly use an anticoagulant:

- Take it *exactly* as prescribed.
- Never double one dose because you missed another. It could cause bleeding. Report missed doses to your doctor.
- Tell all medical personnel you go to that you are taking anticoagulants.
- Don't start or stop any other medicine (including over-the-counter drugs) before checking with your doctor or pharmacist.
- Carry identification that states you are taking anticoagulants.

(continued)

Drugs That Prevent Strokes—Continued

Generic Name/ Brand Name	How Given	Benefits and Uses	Side Effects	Interactions/ Precautions
Coumarin—Continued			• swelling of face, feet, or lower legs • unusual tiredness or weakness • unusual weight gain • yellowing of eyes or skin • diarrhea • nausea • vomiting • skin rash • hives or itching • stomach cramps or pain	• Avoid physical activities that could cause injuries, falls or blows to the body or head. They could cause internal bleeding. • Try to avoid cutting yourself shaving, flossing teeth, etc. • Don't drink alcohol on a daily basis, or take more than 1 or 2 drinks at a time. Alcohol changes the way anticoagulants affect your body. • Eat a normal, balanced diet. If you go on a special diet or are unable to eat for several days (because of stomach upset), check with your doctor.
Heparin Common brand names: Liquaemin Calciparine	Available by prescription only; given by injection	Heparin is an *anticoagulant.*	Heparin, like coumarin anticoagulants, can also cause you to bleed too easily. (See above for the signs outside and inside	Before taking heparin, make sure your doctor knows if you are: • allergic to heparin, beef or pork

your body that unusual bleeding may be occurring. Report them to your doctor immediately.) Check with your doctor as soon as possible if you experience any of these infrequent or rare side effects:

- back or rib pain (long-term use)
- changes in skin color, especially near the place of injection or in the fingers, toes, arms or legs
- chest pain
- chills or fever
- collection of blood under skin (blood blister) at the place of injection
- decrease in height (long-term use)
- frequent or persistent erection
- numbness or tingling in hands or feet
- pain or irritation at place of injection
- pain in arms or legs

- on any special diet, or allergic to any substance
- suffering from any other medical problems
- pregnant or nursing
- a tobacco smoker
- taking any medicines
- recovering from or have recently had any of the following:
  —falls or blows to body or head
  —heavy or unusual menstrual bleeding
  —insertion of an intrauterine device (IUD)
  —medical or dental surgery
  —spinal anesthesia
  —x-ray treatment

Here's how to properly use heparin:

- Take it *exactly* as prescribed.
- Make sure your doctor checks your blood clotting time on a regular basis.

(continued)

Drugs That Prevent Strokes—Continued

Generic Name/ Brand Name	How Given	Benefits and Uses	Side Effects	Interactions/ Precautions
Heparin—Continued			• peeling of skin at place of injection • shortness of breath, troubled breathing or tightness in chest • skin rash, itching or hives • unusual hair loss (long-term use) • unusual runny nose	• Never double one dose if you missed another. It could cause bleeding. (Report missed doses to your doctor.) • Do not take aspirin or any drug containing aspirin while on heparin. • Tell all medical personnel you go to that you use heparin. • Carry identification stating that you are using heparin. • Avoid physical activities that could cause injuries. • Try to avoid cutting yourself while brushing teeth or shaving.

ADAPTED FROM: *Physicians' Desk Reference*, 42nd ed. (Oradell, N.J.: Medical Economics, 1988).

U.S. Pharmacopeia. Drug Information for the Consumer (Rockville, Md.: The United States Pharmacopeial Convention, 1987).

Mark L. Dyken, M.D., chairman, Department of Neurology, Indiana University.

Another group that may be given anticoagulants is people with atrial fibrillation, a condition in which the heart quivers instead of beating regularly. When it does that, blood isn't completely pumped out of the heart's upper chambers, and what remains tends to clot. People with atrial fibrillation are six to eight times more likely than other people to have a stroke because the clots that form can travel to the brain. Yet some reports indicate that the administration of anticoagulants may markedly reduce the risk of stroke in these people.

Anticoagulants can reduce the risk of stroke in people with irregular heartbeats.

But should all people with atrial fibrillation be treated with anticoagulants? Doctors are hesitant to say because of all the risks that accompany these drugs. So Dr. Hart and several others are trying to answer the question in studies where people with atrial fibrillation are given either anticoagulants or aspirin to see if *either* drug will help reduce the number of strokes they suffer. The results will then be compared to a group of people who take no drugs at all.

One of the biggest controversies today is how doctors decide whether to treat the stroke-prone with drugs or surgery. Let's go to the next chapter to examine that controversy and discuss the kinds of surgical techniques doctors have devised to treat those at risk of stroke.

Chapter 8

Preventing Strokes through Surgery

The two surgical procedures doctors have performed in recent years to prevent strokes seem like remarkably straightforward solutions to the problem. If an artery supplying the brain with blood becomes blocked or clogged due to atherosclerosis, then why not remove the blockage, as does one operation called a *carotid endarterectomy*? Or why not reroute blood through other supply routes as does another operation called *extracranial/intracranial bypass*?

Of course, neither operation is simple. Each is a complex procedure with its own risks. The decisions about when, on whom and by whom they should be performed are incredibly difficult. And those decisions have become more difficult in recent years, as many doctors have come to believe that it's often as effective—and much safer—to treat people at risk for stroke with medicines and lifestyle changes. In fact many prominent experts in the stroke field worry that too many of these operations have been performed unnecessarily, at

When surgery does and does not prevent strokes.

too high a risk to the patient. So let's take a look at when surgery does—and does not—prevent strokes.

Do Your Arteries Need a Clean-Out?

Take your hand and feel the pulse in the artery on either side of your neck very, very gently. (Do not compress!) That artery, the carotid, is your main lifeline. Your life depends on an adequate supply of the oxygen in your blood getting through this artery to your brain from minute to minute.

A carotid endarterectomy allows doctors to surgically open up a carotid artery and scrape out the life-threatening fatty buildup caused by atherosclerosis. Since the buildup, called plaque, can eventually block blood flow to the brain, it seems to make sense that removing it would reduce your risk of having a stroke.

The carotid arteries are prime targets for blockages because atherosclerotic buildup occurs most often where blood vessels narrow and branch off. And there's a lot of that going on in your carotids. You have two carotid arteries—one on either side of your neck, each of which divides into two more arteries, the external and internal carotids. The external carotids branch off to another part of your head, while the internal carotids shoot up to the optic nerve and the retina, passing to and through a "traffic circle" in the base of your skull before entering your brain. Both internal and external carotids contribute to this circle.

If you've experienced a transient ischemic attack (TIA), those strokelike attacks that mean you're at high risk for a stroke, one of the first things your doctor will do is check your carotid arteries for evidence of atherosclerotic blockages. A simple way doctors do this is by listening with a stethoscope at your neck for a sound called a bruit.

A carotid endarterectomy is the surgical equivalent of a Roto-Rooter clean-out.

Noisy arteries can "tell" your doctor that they may be clogged.

If a bruit is detected and your doctor suspects your artery is clogged, he would be likely to order an ultrasound scan. This is a very safe procedure that uses sound waves instead of x-ray.

Listening for bruits is also often a part of a routine physical exam, so your doctor could pick up a signal that your arteries may be clogged *before* you have a TIA, too. But don't think you need to go out and get a carotid endarterectomy if your doctor detects a bruit in your neck. Chances are that, unless tests confirm that the artery is dangerously clogged, or unless you have experienced a TIA, most experts would not recommend surgery for you.

Concerns about exactly when carotid endarterectomies *should* be performed, however, are legion. For starters, the number of these operations performed in the United States has grown enormously. Since 1971, there has been an increase of more than 500 percent, according to James C. Grotta, M.D., a neurologist at the University of Texas Medical School who authored a recent review of current medical and surgical therapies being used on people with stroke-related disease. In fact, the National Center for Health Statistics reports that 107,000 people had carotid endarterectomies in 1985—the most recent year for which statistics are available.

Cleaning out neck arteries has increased 500 percent since 1971.

These numbers are enormous compared to the rates of this surgery in places like England, Wales and Canada. In 1984, for example, 433 carotid endarterectomies were performed per million people in the United States, while in England, only 20 operations were performed per million. Yet these two countries have essentially the same incidence of stroke, according to Mark L. Dyken, M.D., chairman of the Department of Neurology at Indiana University, and past chairman of the Stroke Council of the American Heart Association. So the obvious question is—do we know whether these operations truly help to prevent strokes?

Since at least 25 to 50 percent of carotid endarterectomies, according to some studies, are being performed on people who haven't even shown definite symptoms that they're at high risk of a stroke, the answer may be no.

Twenty-five to 50 percent of these operations are performed on people who don't have any symptoms.

And, as if that weren't enough to make you think twice about the operation, there's also evidence from studies that the surgeons who are performing them have an enormously wide range of complication rates—the most significant complications being stroke or death. In fact, a national survey of hospital patients showed that nearly 3 percent of those who undergo carotid endarterectomies die *before they leave the hospital.* So, since most studies have shown that one to five times as many have strokes as die, it is possible that 10 percent or more of all people who have a carotid endarterectomy will die or suffer a debilitating stroke within 30 days of the operation.

These frightening statistics have caused the surgeons who perform these operations to select their patients more carefully. And, according to several surgeons we consulted, many are now calling for stricter monitoring procedures that would make their colleagues keep better records of their complication rates.

Now doctors are selecting their patients more carefully.

So who should—and should not—have a carotid endarterectomy?

There are two important groups to consider when answering that question—those with stroke symptoms who have evidence of a clogged artery, and those with a clogged artery who've had no symptoms that a stroke may be imminent.

Surgery for Symptoms? It Depends

You might be a candidate for surgery if blocked arteries caused a TIA.

Doctors who treat the stroke-prone are in much greater agreement on when to consider surgery on people who've had definite symptoms because these people are more clearly at risk. The most definite symptom would be a TIA, which temporarily causes numbness on one side of your body, slurred speech and other symptoms. When a TIA occurs in someone as a result of a serious carotid artery blockage (doctors call this blockage a *stenosis*), that's when surgeons might act.

How do doctors know if a blocked artery is to blame for your TIA? They can tell which parts of the brain were cut off from their blood supply by the strokelike symptoms you have. If you had a weakness on the right side of your body, for example, doctors would suspect that it was the carotid artery supplying blood to the left side of your brain that was to blame.

"If a patient has a single TIA and a carotid artery with under 80 percent stenosis [blockage], I would try treating this person with aspirin to see if that stopped the TIA from recurring," says Richard F. Kempczinski, M.D., a vascular surgeon at the University of Cincinnati College of Medicine. And, since aspirin has been shown to reduce the risk of stroke in people who've experienced TIAs, Stuart Myers, M.D., a vascular surgeon at the University of Texas Health Science Center, agrees.

Aspirin might make the surgery unnecessary.

If there is a recurrence of TIA symptoms, however, or if the carotid artery looks like it is more than 80 percent blocked, both surgeons say they would then suggest an arteriogram, an invasive test which gives a much more accurate picture of the extent of the blockage. Arteriograms are performed only on people who are being considered for surgery, since this test itself carries a very small risk of causing a stroke or death.

An arteriogram can help doctors decide.

If the arteriogram confirmed a high degree of blockage and aspirin therapy was ineffective in stopping the TIAs, both surgeons say they would recommend surgery.

Someone who has experienced a TIA caused by a carotid artery blocked 75 percent or more is at a very high risk for a subsequent stroke, says Wesley Moore, M.D., chief of vascular surgery at the

A good surgeon can unclog your arteries.

University of California in Los Angeles (UCLA). "The risk is close to 10 percent within the first year and 6 percent each year thereafter, for a combined 35 percent stroke risk within five years of the TIA," he says. "In the hands of a good surgeon, the blockage can be removed without the operation causing the patient to have a stroke. And the risk of a subsequent stroke related to the artery operated on is reduced to one half of 1 percent per year."

Of course, you could still have a stroke related to the other carotid artery in your neck, or for another reason, says Dr. Moore. That's why doctors monitor patients closely after it's been discovered that they have a severe blockage. "Thirty to 40 percent of those with stenosis on one side will come up with a blockage on the other side," he estimates. It's a signal that they're vulnerable to atherosclerotic disease.

If you've already had a stroke and your arteries are blocked, surgery may reduce your risk of a second stroke.

Besides operating on patients with recurrent TIAs, the surgeons we interviewed also said they would consider operating on someone with a severe blockage who had also recovered well from a mild stroke. (Those who haven't recovered well are at too high a risk.) "That person has an even greater risk of another stroke than someone with a TIA—a risk of about 9 percent per year," says Dr. Moore. "And a successful operation can reduce that risk to about 2 percent a year."

Although the surgical community seems to strongly feel that carotid endarterectomies are warranted on the kinds of patients we've just described, many experts would still like to see those beliefs supported by a well-designed study.

Just such a study—involving two groups of people with severely blocked arteries who've experienced TIAs—has been recently funded by the National Institutes of Health and is being organized and run by some of the same researchers who proved the ineffectiveness of another operation previously used to prevent strokes.

The new study, which will not be concluded until well into the next decade, will include some 3,000 people who will be followed for up to seven years, according to University of Western Ontario neurologist Vladimir C. Hachinski, M.D., one of the study's investigators. All the study participants will get the best medical care and half of them will be randomly assigned to receive carotid endarterectomies. If the operation is effective, the people who are operated on will have significantly fewer strokes and deaths than the "control" group which didn't have surgery, according to Dr. Hachinski. If the operation is ineffective, the number of strokes and deaths in both groups will be relatively equal.

Still, some surgeons believe so strongly that carotid endarterectomies are warranted in TIA patients with severe blockage that they don't believe the study is going to tell them anything they don't already know. "Most of us don't feel it's an open question," says Dr. Moore. "As long as you've got a good surgeon with low complication rates, you're going to benefit."

Their faith is apparently sustained by a study of people who experienced TIAs during the 1960s, says Dr. Moore. Half of the study's participants received carotid endarterectomies, but because the rate of strokes or death from the surgery itself was so high, it cancelled out any benefit. In patients who didn't have a stroke or die from the surgery, however, their risk of stroke was just 4 percent after three and a half years of follow-up. The other half of the study's participants had a 12 percent risk.

The new National Institutes of Health study may yield better results, since surgeons now believe they can do the operation with much lower complication rates—thanks to better surgical techniques.

Surgery for People with No Symptoms

But what about patients who have blockages in carotid arteries without having had TIAs or other symptoms of stroke?

It's in trying to decide who among this group should have surgery that debate rages fiercely among various members of the medical and surgical community. Neurologists (medical doctors who specialize in the brain) and neurosurgeons (doctors who specialize in brain surgery) tend to be conservative.

"I don't have any of my asymptomatic [without symptoms] patients operated on," says Dr. Dyken.

No symptoms, no surgery, says one neurologist.

Adds John R. Little, M.D., a neurosurgeon who heads the Cerebrovascular Surgery Section at the Cleveland Clinic Foundation, "I would tend not to operate on asymptomatic patients unless they had a very severe stenosis—more than 90 percent narrowing—and they were under age 70. In addition, they would have to be relatively healthy, and without major heart disease before I would operate." Unfortunately, heart problems are common in people who have clogged carotid arteries.

Vascular surgeons, who specialize in operating on blood vessels, tend to be more liberal. Many vascular surgeons recommend the operation for asymptomatic people who have more than 80 percent of a carotid artery blocked, says Dr. Moore, because they believe that these people are at much higher risk of stroke than the general population. Dr. Myers, also a vascular surgeon, agrees that he would consider surgery in these patients, if there was evidence that the artery was getting progressively more clogged and if they were healthy and free of serious heart disease.

Dr. Moore acknowledges, however, that despite suggestive evidence, it's never been adequately proven that carotid endarterectomies help reduce stroke risk in people with blocked arteries but no symptoms. And, for that reason, he's one of the surgeons involved in another National Institutes of Health study which will divide 1,500 people with blocked arteries but no symptoms of stroke into two groups, half of whom will get carotid endarterectomies. All the patients will receive aspirin as well and they'll be followed for up to five years to see which of them develop strokes. If carotid endarterectomies are worthwhile, the group that gets them should have fewer strokes than the group that does not.

There's no proof that surgery will help.

A similar study, this one being conducted by ten Veterans Administration Medical Centers, will recruit 500 patients with blocked arteries but no symptoms to be studied for five years. Again, participants will be divided into two groups. One group will have carotid endarterectomies, and the number of strokes in both groups will be carefully tabulated.

But the question of whether these operations truly reduce your risk of stroke isn't the only reason the wisdom of carotid endarterectomies for people without symptoms is so hotly debated. While most people who have blocked arteries but no symptoms have a very low risk of having a stroke without a warning like a TIA, the surgeons who often perform these operations can have very high complication rates—sometimes much higher than the risk of stroke without the operation.

A bad surgeon can increase your risk of stroke.

A study performed by researchers at the University of Cincinnati, including Dr. Kempczinski, found that in a year's worth of carotid endarterectomies, there was a 5.3 percent chance of surgery-associated stroke or death in patients with no symptoms. The surgery actually *doubled* the risk of stroke and death. And many doctors fear the rate may be higher than that among less-skilled surgeons than the ones who were studied. A review of 1,302 carotid endarterectomies by the

An individual surgeon's rate of complications can range from 0 to 21 percent.

Rand Corporation, for example, reveals that complication rates range from 0 to 21 percent.

This kind of evidence led Anthony J. Furlan, M.D., director of the Cleveland Clinic's Cerebrovascular Program, to recently tell doctors that he never sends asymptomatic patients to a surgeon unless the surgeon's rate of operation-associated strokes and/or deaths is less than 2 percent.

A surgeon's complication rate should be less than 2 percent, says one neurologist.

Think that's impossible? UCLA's Dr. Moore, for example, says that in records they kept for asymptomatic patients operated on between 1980 and 1984, the risk of stroke or death at the time of the operation was only 0.6 percent. And by 1987, none had experienced strokes stemming from the artery that surgeons operated on. So it's possible interestingly, the Rand Corporation study confirms that academic medical centers have significantly lower complication rates than community hospitals.

Academic medical centers have lower complication rates than community hospitals.

What's the bottom line? Get a recommendation by your doctor and/or a neurologist that in his opinion you truly need the operation *before* you're referred to a surgeon, says Dr. Little—whether you've experienced a TIA or not.

Whom Do You Trust?

A referring doctor or neurologist can also be an invaluable help in finding a surgeon with low complication rates. "Your doctor should have tremendous confidence in the surgeon he's recommending and he should know the complication rate of that surgeon," says Dr. Myers. And you should feel perfectly comfortable asking your doctor the complication rates of any surgeon he recommends.

Ask your doctor the complication rate of any surgeon he recommends.

Once you're sitting in the surgeon's office, you should also ask how many carotid endarterectomies he's performed and how often he currently performs them.

Your surgeon should be experienced at doing the operation and he should be performing it on a regular basis, says Dr. Kempczinski. "If his total experience is 200 to 300 of these operations, that's a great number," says Dr. Moore. "On the other hand, if he's done only 10, I'd be hestitant." Dr. Moore also advises against any surgeon who is doing fewer than 12 carotid endarterectomies per year. "Under that number," he says, "I'd be concerned."

Don't use any surgeon who performs less than 12 operations a year, one doctor advises.

You should also ascertain that he's a board-certified surgeon who has had special training in performing carotid endarterectomies during his residency, adds Dr. Kempczinski. Ask to see his certification. If you're referred to a general surgeon, ask him if he's had any special training in operating on blood vessels, advises Dr. Moore.

Then, the most important question of all: What are his personal complication rates for carotid endarterectomies? An acceptable rate of complications (including both strokes and deaths) from this surgery is 3 percent among people who had a blocked artery but no symptoms, agree Drs. Moore and Kempczinski. After all, if you fit this description, your risk of a stroke *without* surgery is probably about 3 percent—so you should never agree to surgery by a doctor whose technique causes stroke or death in *more* than 3 percent of his patients.

Among people the surgeon has operated on who have experienced TIAs (and are therefore at greater risk of a stroke—10 percent the first year after a TIA and 6 percent after that), 6 percent should be the upper limit of complications from the surgery, believes Dr. Moore. And, among patients who've had a prior stroke and are at even higher risk of a stroke (about 9 percent a year), the complication rate limit should be no higher than 7 percent.

While doctors agree that surgeons' complication rates should certainly not be higher than the figures we've just cited, some doctors feel that you should not consider surgery with a doctor who has a complication rate over 3 percent for *all* his patients—including those who've experienced TIA's

Some doctors feel any complication rate over 3 percent is too high.

or minor strokes. This is an issue you'll have to discuss with your own doctor.

In any case, "The surgeon should have his complication rates on the tips of his fingers," says Dr. Moore. "If he doesn't, it means he either hasn't kept track of them or he does it too infrequently."

Dr. Kempczinski agrees. "He should be able to give you a real review of his records. For example: 'I have done 150 of these operations, and I followed all of my patients for five years afterward and found . . . .' "

Both surgeons warn that your surgeon should be telling you his own *personal* results—not the success rates for carotid endarterectomies that he cites from studies of others who've performed the operation. Some studies show *very* low complication rates—rates that a particular surgeon may not be able to duplicate.

If the surgeon is uncomfortable or can't answer your questions when you ask for numbers, go elsewhere, says Dr. Moore.

As a general rule, you're more likely to find surgeons who are keeping track of their numbers at larger, university medical centers, adds Dr. Kempczinski. Although many surgeons at smaller community hospitals are now doing a good job of tracking their results. "Quality assurance programs at hospitals are making both hospitals and doctors more accountable for the procedures they perform, so this should help patients who are looking for numbers," says Dr. Little.

Once you know the risks—both of having the operation and not having it—you and your family can make an informed decision that will send you back out into the world, or into the operating room, confident that you made the right choice.

A Good Idea that Didn't Work

The extracranial/intracranial (EC/IC) bypass operation allows surgeons to take a healthy scalp artery on top of the head (*extracranial* means outside the

Avoid any surgeon who can't give you numbers.

Knowing the risks will give you confidence in your choice.

skull) and pass it through a hole in the skull where it is connected to an artery inside the brain (*intra-cranial*). This brings blood flow back to a part of the brain that was being choked off by a clogged artery by "bypassing" that blockage.

When EC/IC bypass surgery was at the height of its popularity, literally dozens of studies showed that the operation helped restore blood flow—and the life-sustaining nutrients that blood supplies—to parts of the brain that needed it. But no one knew for sure whether the procedure would actually prevent stroke.

A surgical bypass could restore blood flow, studies reported.

Finally a distinguished group of neurologists, neurosurgeons and neuroradiologists (all special-ists in how the brain operates) decided to study a large group of people, all of whom were potential candidates for a bypass operation. To be eligible, the participants had to have symptoms that indi-cate a stroke was likely to occur or to have sus-tained a minor stroke. They also had to show evi-dence that an artery inside the brain—the middle cerebral artery—or a carotid artery was almost completely blocked by atherosclerotic buildup.

Then, with the participants' consent and un-derstanding, the researchers, who were called the EC/IC Bypass Study Group, randomly assigned them either to have bypass surgery or to forgo it. The two groups were carefully matched in size, age, sex, other stroke risk factors (like high blood pressure and heart disease) and by where and how much an artery was clogged. All the participants were also given aspirin, if they could tolerate it, since aspirin has been shown to reduce stroke risk.

A study to find the truth.

Almost 1,400 people were recruited from medical centers in North America, Europe and Asia and monitored from two to seven years to see if the operation would help reduce the number of people who suffered strokes or died of stroke-re-lated causes.

What the researchers found is that the group which underwent surgery actually had *more* fatal

How to Prepare for Surgery

Preparing your body and mind for surgery is probably as important as all those presurgery tests you're being asked to take. Studies have shown that people who are prepared have swifter recoveries and fewer complications. So, if it looks like stroke prevention surgery is in the near future for you, take the following precautions.

Eat well. A good diet, high in vitamins and minerals, should be one of your priorities before surgery. There's a tremendous amount of stress on major organ functions when you're recovering from surgery, according to James L. Mullen, M.D., of the Hospital of the University of Pennsylvania. Your body needs all the nutrients it can get to handle the shock of an operation.

The most important nutrients in terms of wound healing and infection fighting are vitamins A and C and the mineral zinc. Best food sources: yellow and orange vegetables and fruits, green leafy vegetables and liver for vitamin A; green peppers, citrus fruits, broccoli, brussels sprouts and cantaloupe for vitamin C; and beef, lamb, chicken, oysters, cheese and pumpkin seeds for zinc.

Be informed. One of the most important ways you can prepare for surgery is to get as much information about the procedure as you can. Studies show that patients who know a lot about what's going to happen recover faster and experience less pain after surgery. Many hospitals are now providing informational programs for surgery patients, so be sure to inquire about them. Your doctor may also be able to recommend read-

A surgical bypass actually seems to cause the deaths and strokes it's supposed to prevent.

and nonfatal strokes—and they occurred sooner—than the group that had no surgery. This held true even after the researchers took into account the patients' age, sex, other stroke risk factors and the type and extent of their clogged arter-

ing materials. But if explicit details about the surgery make you feel uncomfortable, according to the late Emily Mumford, Ph.D., a professor at Columbia College of Physicians and Surgeons, stop when you've learned enough.

Deal with preoperative stress. The chemicals released by your body when it's under stress can actually affect your recovery. So your hospital may have a special stress-reduction program for surgery patients. If it doesn't, there's a highly effective two-volume tape set you can order. Called "Successful Surgery and Recovery," it's authored by Emmett Miller, M.D., a respected stress-reduction expert.

The first tape, which is meant to be listened to preoperatively, begins with a progressive relaxation exercise that reminds you to concentrate on the time beyond your surgery when you'll feel strong and healthy again. This "think positive" approach gets you beyond the negative feelings you may be having about undergoing surgery and actually helps program your body for a successful recovery. The second half of this tape walks you through the sequence of surgery so you know what to expect, and it also contains suggestions for how to relax so you'll get a good night's sleep before the operation.

The second tape helps people who are recovering from surgery and experiencing pain. The tapes can be purchased as a set for $15.95 from Emmett Miller, M.D., P.O. Box W, Stanford, CA 94309.

ies—all of which could affect who developed strokes. The operation did help reduce the number of transient ischemic attacks suffered by patients who were operated on—but those *not* operated on enjoyed just about the same reduction.

Most of the operations were successful in that the neurosurgeons were able to safely graft the outside skull artery to the artery inside the brain and get blood flowing through. Clearly they shunted more blood to the brain but did not improve brain function. So the failure of the bypass to reduce strokes can't be explained away by poor surgical technique or ability, the study also pointed out.

The results of this landmark study caused a dramatic change in the number of bypass operations performed in the United States. "I only do one or two a year now in patients who fail even the best medical therapy," says Dr. Little. "I used to average about 30 a year."

But why, if the results of this study were so clearcut, are surgeons performing any at all? Some critics say that because the study was so large, it may have missed subgroups of patients who might still benefit from the procedure.

Some doctors still recommend a bypass.

"We can't say that [absolutely] no one would profit from a bypass, based on the results of this study," says Dr. Hachinski, a participating neurologist in the study. "It's not right to use the results to generalize to all. However, the burden of proof is now on those who still believe it works to find out who it will help.

"Our study should not prohibit doctors from performing bypass surgery or seeing a role for it if they believe in individual cases that it will help," says Dr. Hachinski.

A bypass may help if you meet four specific criteria, one doctor says.

What might some of those cases be? Dr. Little says that he would consider bypass surgery for someone under the following conditions: (1) the person had a totally blocked carotid artery; (2) the artery could not be surgically cleaned out by a carotid endarterectomy; (3) the person was having TIA symptoms or had experienced a minor stroke; and (4) aspirin and anticoagulants had not worked to prevent stroke symptoms from recurring.

Dr. Hachinski says someone who had a giant aneurysm—or hernia—in a brain blood vessel might also be an acceptable candidate.

So will an EC/IC bypass help *you?* Only your doctor can say. But if you don't fit the very narrow profile described here by the top stroke doctors   **Think.**
from around the country, think twice about accepting anyone's recommendations for surgery.

Part **3**

Regenerating the Mind, the Body, the Spirit

Chapter 9

The Brave New World of Stroke Rehabilitation

When Ed, a stroke survivor in his late sixties, entered the Lourdes Regional Rehabilitation Center at Our Lady of Lourdes Medical Center in Camden, New Jersey, he had trouble sitting in a wheelchair. A large white sheet—folded in thirds like a diaper and tied around his hips and the wheelchair—kept him from sliding out.

Not that he was planning to travel. He couldn't see anything on his left, didn't know his left side even existed and couldn't begin to make the chair go where he wanted it to anyway. In fact Ed was completely dependent on those around him. It took two nurses just to get him to the bathroom.

With time and therapy during a five-week stay at Lourdes, however, Ed learned how to recognize when he was sliding out of his wheelchair so that he could put on the brakes and push himself back up. Intensive physical therapy taught him to steer the wheelchair with his right foot and hand. Therapists also helped him compensate for vision problems by training him to turn his whole head to the left to see what was going on over there. He also learned how to transfer himself from bed to chair to bathroom with minimal assistance.

Because of these strides, Ed regained his independence. He was able to go home to live with his wife, Ann, who—also trained by the Lourdes therapists—could provide the small amounts of help he needed. This was critically important to Ed because, as he told the therapists, "I don't want to be a burden. And I don't like asking for a lot of help."

Rehabilitation may be the key to independence.

Maybe Ed's body would have naturally recovered some of the function that he had lost when he suffered his stroke. It often does. But, without therapy, who would have given him the expert help in learning the best and easiest ways to transfer from bed to chair or use a wheelchair with only one hand and foot? Who would have taught him the best ways to compensate for his left-side neglect? Who would have helped him maintain his muscle tone and strength to achieve their highest potential?

Your body can sometimes recover without any help at all.

Though it's impossible to say for sure, it's a good bet that without the help of the Lourdes program, Ed might be in a nursing home today—separated from his wife because she couldn't possibly provide the help he would need to perform just the most rudimentary activities of life: eating, getting around and going to the bathroom. And that would be a tragedy.

But rehab can frequently mean the difference between a nursing home and home.

Given stories like Ed's—and therapists all over the country can tell you countless others like his—it seems hard to believe that there is any argument against sending stroke survivors to comprehensive rehabilitation programs. And yet, some medical professionals are still skeptical about the benefits of rehabilitation.

The crux of the argument, some doctors say, is that no really good scientific study has been able to prove that rehabilitation therapy helps the brain recover any more than it would have on its own. If a person is going to recover the use of his leg, for example, it will happen if his brain is capable of making it happen. Not because of a rehabilitation program.

But rehabilitation specialists (called doctors of physical medicine and rehabilitation, or physiatrists) say doctors who think that way are missing a big part of the reason for rehabilitation.

Physiatrists focus on the larger picture, seeing brain recovery as only one part of the recovery process for a stroke survivor. "We look at their ability to care for themselves, to move around on their own, to feel independent again," says Thomas P. Anderson, M.D., senior physiatrist at Spaulding Rehabilitation Hospital in Boston. And as Ed and millions of others prove every day—you don't have to recover the use of your leg or arm to be independent.

Fostering independence in a motivational atmosphere that focuses on practical ways to improve a stroke survivor's quality of life, using whatever abilities he still has—that's what good stroke rehabilitation programs are all about, says Dr. Anderson, who wrote the chapter on stroke for the medical world's "bible" on rehabilitation.

Using what you have is what it's all about.

But the freedom of each stroke survivor's life is not the only issue at stake. There's also a tremendous financial argument for rehabilitating stroke survivors like Ed so that they can live independently.

Studies show that once they survive the first few months of high death rates (25 percent), stroke survivors live at least seven years or longer after their strokes. And the cost of long-term nursing home care for that period of time far exceeds the cost of rehabilitation. "If patients can be discharged to their own homes instead of confined to institutions, rehabilitation quickly pays for itself," say experts at the Mayo Clinic. "It is cost-effective to help totally dependent survivors become even partially self-sufficient."

Rehab costs less than a nursing home.

Are there any stroke survivors who would *not* benefit from a stroke rehabilitation program? Some doctors believe that there are probably two groups at either end of the spectrum of stroke survivors who do not need or would not benefit from a program. The first group is those who will get better quickly on their own. The second group is those who will never get better no matter what efforts are made. But in the middle is a third group of people who are probably better served by rehabilitation.

Unfortunately, no one has come up with a way to identify the dividing lines between these three groups, says neurologist Philip A. Wolf, M.D., the principal stroke scientist for the Framingham Heart Study, a long-running population study of over 5,000 residents of Framingham, Massachusetts. So it's difficult to predict in the immediate post-stroke period which patients will benefit from a rehabilitation program—either in the short- or long-term.

But there *are* several factors unrelated to the kind of stroke injury the patient sustained which doctors know can influence how much a rehabilitation program will help a survivor and whether the gains can be sustained, says Dr. Anderson. Many survivors, once out of the motivational atmosphere of a rehab center, lose the incentive to keep doing the independent tasks they learned there. That's why one of the most important factors for continuing success seems to be a strong, supportive family.

A strong, supportive family is the key to successful rehab.

A study performed at the Burke Rehabilitation Center in White Plains, New York, found that patients sustained the impressive gains in mobility and in performing the activities of daily living—dressing, toileting and eating, for example—that they had made at Burke for up to two years after their stays. And the crucial element was their families, whom Burke trains to be active participants in survivors' therapy and exercise programs. Those patients whose families remained most involved in

And successful rehab is more likely to be sustained by an actively involved family.

their therapy after they left the hospital were most likely to have sustained the gains made at Burke.

"The family has to know how to manage the stroke survivor," says Michael J. Reding, M.D., attending physician at Burke and leading author on the study. "Most rehabilitation centers see that as a crucial aspect of successful aftercare."

"If we know that the family is there, willing and able to help take care of a survivor—that's a critical factor in deciding on our goals for him," says Charles Norelli, M.D., staff physiatrist, Good Shepherd Rehabilitation Hospital, Allentown, Pennsylvania. "He may not need to walk or become totally independent to go home. Getting him out of bed and into a wheelchair may be enough. If he can do that, given his family support, he's a good candidate for rehabilitation."

Another factor that influences how much a rehab program can help is whether it's conducted at an inpatient center or an outpatient facility. There are four separate studies which show that stroke survivors make more strides in the inpatient stroke unit at a rehabilitation center, says Dr. Reding, than those who receive rehabilitation as outpatients or in a less-coordinated fashion.

Inpatient rehabilitation seems to be more successful than using an outpatient facility.

The reason? A coordinated team of stroke rehabilitation specialists, headed by a physican who is well-trained in rehabilitation, is an absolutely crucial aspect of good programs, adds Dr. Anderson. And it's most readily accessible at an inpatient facility. Ideally, the stroke team physician should be a physiatrist, but internists, family physicians, neurologists and other doctors have also successfully headed up stroke rehabilitation teams. If other doctors do lead the group, however, they should be experienced and knowledgeable about stroke rehabilitation.

A team of rehab specialists, coordinated by a physiatrist, may be the ideal approach.

Stroke survivors and their families should demand a team-approach rehabilitation program coordinated and headed by a physician because without this, "It's not real rehabilitation," says Dr.

A single doctor who coordinates the team's efforts is imperative.

(continued on page 196)

How to Choose a Rehabilitation Center

What should you look for in a rehabilitation facility? Here are some tips based on advice from the American Hospital Association, the National Association of Rehabilitation Facilities, and the Commission on Accreditation of Rehabilitation Facilities (CARF), as well as other experts in stroke care whom we consulted.

Accreditation. The rehabilitation facility should be accredited by CARF and/or the Joint Commission on Accreditation of Healthcare Organizations. Ask how long the center has been accredited and when accreditation ends since accreditation is renewed based on periodic reinspections. If a center is accredited by either or both of these organizations, it has to meet high standards of care.

Staffing. Are the medical doctors physiatrists (doctors of physical medicine and rehabilitation) or doctors with rehabilitation experience? It's critical that doctors experienced in rehabilitation head up rehabilitation programs. The facility should also have access to other consulting doctors in related areas in case a stroke survivor should need those services (neurologists, internists, heart specialists, etc.).

Services. The rehabilitation center should offer a wide array of services, including physical, occupational, speech, language, hearing and recreational therapy; social and psychological counseling; and vocational services. In addition, the center should be able to fit its patients for various braces and other equipment used by the stroke-impaired.

Other special programs. Look for centers that offer special programs that could be particularly helpful for the stroke survivor—work adjustment and skills training (if he is returning to work), outpatient programs (if the survivor will need therapy after a stay at the center), stroke support groups for the survivor and family (these win high marks from stroke survivors and their families and seem to be much needed by them), driver education programs for the disabled, sexuality education and counseling, dental care, athletic programs (wheelchair sports and swimming, for example) and home health services (they may be able to help coordinate the services you'll need when the survivor returns home).

Equipment and accessibility. Does the center have a full array of wheelchairs and other equipment that survivors can use and try out while they're there? Are there training areas that simulate kitchens, bathrooms, bedrooms and cars so survivors can practice daily living skills? Is there real access for stroke-impaired people to all areas in the rehabilitation center—including bathrooms, grounds, parking lots, elevators, etc.?

Coordination of care. There should be a team of rehabilitation specialists caring for the stroke survivor. The care should be coordinated and the team should be headed by a physician—preferably a physiatrist. Does the stroke rehabilitation team meet often, preferably once a week, to report on the survivor's progress in each area so they can further coordinate their efforts? These are essential points, since without this coordination it's not real rehabilitation. The survivors themselves and/or their families should be periodically included in team conferences.

Planning for homecoming. The facility should be able to help you plan a care program for the stroke survivor after he leaves the rehabilitation center. The stroke team should be able to help assess your home for changes that need to be made and they should encourage trial home visits for the stroke survivor so that problems or questions can be resolved before the final return home.

They should also include families in therapy sessions so that the caregivers can learn techniques for home care. Supportive families are a critical

(continued)

How to Choose
a Rehabilitation Center—
Continued

factor in how well survivors fare after they return home. Facilities should also be able to systematically refer survivors and their families to home care agencies and services.

Success rates. These rates vary enormously from one facility to another. So be sure to ask how many patients return home after treatment. Keep in mind, however, that whether a survivor returns home or not, the best measure of a facility's success is if the team met the goals and objectives that were planned for the survivor.

If you are having a problem locating a good rehabilitation facility, you can contact the National Association of Rehabilitation Facilities, P.O. Box 17675, Washington, DC 20041. The organization will send you a list of facilities in a three-state area closest to where you live.

Anderson. "A lot of hospitals are putting in token rehabilitation units, with perhaps a few therapists on staff, but no real coordinated rehabilitation effort." If this is the kind of rehabilitation that's being recommended to you, ask your doctor for some better options. (See the box, "How to Choose a Rehabilitation Center," on page 194.)

But just who are the crucial members of a stroke rehabilitation team? Besides the physician, there should be physical, occupational and speech therapists, rehabilitation nurses, psychologists/psychiatrists, social workers and recreational therapists. Vocational counselors should also be available if the stroke survivor wants to return to work. Dieticians should also be available to advise the team if the survivor has problems with eating or

The rehab team should meet on a regular basis to discuss the stroke survivor's progress.

other nutritional concerns. And the whole team should meet on a regular basis to discuss each stroke survivor's case and progress so that they can coordinate and complement each others' efforts.

It's this cooperative spirit that makes the stroke team approach so effective. Since every survivor's needs are different, you never know whose services will be needed most. But the combined effort usually gets results. We'll describe the roles of each team member in a moment. But before we do, let's talk for a few minutes about the period just after a stroke, when the stroke survivor is still in a regular hospital.

A cooperative spirit makes the stroke team effective.

When Should Rehabilitation Begin?

Efforts at rehabilitation can and should begin just as soon as doctors are sure that the stroke is complete. In fact without early rehabilitation the stroke survivor is in danger of suffering some common physical and psychological complications that can really slow down his or her rehabilitation. Generally, doctors say, in-hospital rehabilitation efforts should center on physical therapy, bladder and bowel retraining, and mental stimulation.

The earlier the rehabilitation begins, the better.

Nurses and physical therapists, for example, should quickly begin programs to prevent two common complications after a stroke: contractures and bedsores. Contractures—which are literally shortened muscles—occur when unused muscles tighten and prevent a joint from being able to move through it's normal range of motion. The ankle joint, for example, should be able to bend and straighten your foot.

Nurses and physical therapists can prevent contractures by performing gentle, passive range-of-motion exercises especially on the stroke survivor's paralyzed side, if the survivor cannot do so. Of course, if the survivor can exercise, then he should be shown how to do the exercises himself. These should be performed several times daily.

Gentle movement and exercise immediately after a stroke will prevent pain and frozen joints.

What happens if muscles and joints aren't put through their paces? The joint can freeze, leaving the stroke survivor unable to extend his or her arm, for example, at the elbow. The arm would remain in a bent—and often painful—position.

Nurses should also move the survivor often and very carefully position his or her limbs when lying down and sitting up, especially the limbs on the side of the body which is paralyzed. Moving around and good positioning will help to prevent both contractures and bedsores, which are painful skin ulcers caused by lying still for too long.

Another common problem—one that affects the shoulder—is that a paralyzed arm becomes such a "dead weight" it can pull the arm bone, the humerus, out of the shoulder socket. That's why nurses are careful to be sure that the arm is well positioned and supported—using slings, bolsters and other props.

Thirty percent of a stroke survivor's strength is lost if he lies around for even three weeks.

Helping the stroke survivor move about in general is also an extremely important part of recovery because getting muscles to move again helps to keep them functioning. And strong. "About 30 percent of a patient's strength is lost if he or she stays in bed for three weeks," says Michele Miller, R.N., director of rehabilitation nursing at the Lourdes Regional Rehabilitation Center. And moving around also means that nurses and physical therapists can begin teaching survivors how to handle common activities of daily living like transferring from bed to chair. Moreover, keeping stroke survivors physically active is crucial because they're going to need some stamina for the strenuous rehabilitation program to come, says Miller.

A physical therapist can put you on the road to recovery with an initial evaluation.

A physical therapist who visits the stroke survivor in the period immediately after a stroke should perform an evaluation and devise a program for the survivor, says Barbara Freiberg, a licensed physical therapist at North Carolina Baptist Hospital, Winston-Salem, North Carolina.

"I begin by evaluating the patient's range of motion by moving all his joints or getting him to move the ones he can. I note whatever active motion there is on the affected side. Are his muscles flaccid, that is, lacking in tension? What can the muscles do? Do they have any strength?

"Then I check for sensation on the affected side. Can the person feel the difference between sharp and dull objects, between light and deep touch? Can the person tell without looking what object I've placed in his hand? Is the person aware of his arm or leg in space? I usually move an arm or leg and ask the patient to tell me without looking what direction I am moving it.

"I also check the person's coordination—his ability to make smooth movements. Can he pick up small objects or move something from one place to another?" In addition, Freiberg also tests a stroke survivor's reflexes and balance, as well as his ability to walk.

Another crucial part of early rehabilitation is to get survivors going on a program to retrain their bladders and bowels. Many survivors initially have problems in these areas and Miller says families and stroke survivors should push for help in getting the retraining program going as soon as possible. "If a patient still has a catheter [a urine collection device] in, ask why. And how long before it can come out? After all, eventually the patient will have to deal with his bladder and bowels. Why not begin? Put yourself in that person's place. Wouldn't you like to get that under control as soon as possible?"

Early bladder and bowel retraining is important.

See if nurses can begin helping the stroke survivor use a commode instead of a bedpan, since it's a lot easier to void and move bowels there. If the stroke survivor is having trouble controlling his bladder, see if the nursing staff can get him to the bathroom more often—once every two hours instead of once every four hours, says Miller. This kind of "timed voiding" can help the survivor

Timed voiding can help achieve bladder control.

achieve normal bladder control—which a majority of stroke survivors eventually do. A bowel retraining program should also be started as soon as possible, using some of the same concepts.

Stroke survivors also need brief but regular periods of stimulation—people to talk with them so they stay socially involved. This is just as true if the stroke survivor is suffering from some form of communication problem which affects his ability to listen and/or speak.

Talking to stroke survivors will keep them involved and stimulated.

The tendency is to speak to such survivors as if they were children or, worse still, talk about them in the third person even while in their presence. Stroke survivors should be encouraged to try and communicate frequently but briefly in a quiet, low-commotion atmosphere. If communication is a problem, you should make every effort to see that a speech therapist evaluates the survivor as soon as possible so that successful forms of communication can be reestablished. If a stroke survivor cannot speak, for example, or seem to understand what you're saying, he may be able to communicate through gestures and pictures.

Communication is a critical part of stroke recovery.

Even though these early efforts at communication may tire the survivor—and seem fruitless if it doesn't seem as though he is able to understand what's being said—they're nevertheless critical as part of the recovery process, says Dr. Anderson. Otherwise, if a survivor is left alone, his or her personality quickly begins to deteriorate, often contributing to depression which can seriously hinder later efforts at rehabilitation. And when you're depressed, it's a lot harder to motivate yourself to work hard at intensive rehabilitation.

"We who work at rehabilitation centers often have to spend several weeks undoing the unnecessary complications that occur to stroke survivors who were not given early rehabilitation efforts," says Dr. Anderson.

Rehab nurse Michele Miller agrees. But she also points out that the situation at some regular hospitals may not lend itself to early rehabilitation. "Many nurses are not familiar with rehabilitation or how important it is to stroke survivors," says Miller. "You have to remember, a nurse's orientation is toward survival—keeping the patient alive. They may not have the long view that once the patient is medically stable, they should be helped to get on with their lives. Stroke is not an illness, it's a disability—you don't get better by lying there."

> **Make sure the nursing staff understands that the stroke survivor won't get better by just lying in bed.**

In addition, says Miller, nursing shortages across the country have made it difficult to offer the time for the kind of rehabilitation care a stroke survivor needs. Stroke survivors often have urinary catheters in far longer than they need to, for example, because nurses may find this easier and less time consuming than the whole process of bladder retraining.

Another problem is that some hospitals may not have the full range of therapists on their staff to offer the expert help in physical, occupational and speech therapy that should begin as soon as possible.

What it all comes down to, says Miller, is that families of stroke survivors have to be educated consumers, demanding these services from regular hospitals—an idea that Dr. Anderson seconds.

> **Families of stroke survivors have to demand that hospitals provide a full range of therapy services.**

The Stroke Team Goes to Work

When a stroke survivor arrives at a rehabilitation hospital, members of the stroke team evaluate the survivor and form a plan of action, with input from him and his family. Each of the different specialists reports to the team on specific problems the survivor is having, and they work out goals they hope to accomplish with him.

> **The first step in rehab is a plan of action.**

The rehabilitation doctor oversees the whole plan and keeps the team informed on whatever medical problems the survivor may have that would have an impact on rehabilitation efforts.

The rehab nurse organizes a plan for caring for the patient, working on bowel and bladder retraining (if that's still a problem) and reinforcing the therapies the patient is practicing. For that matter, all the members of the stroke team reinforce the efforts of the others. If a survivor is learning to walk, for example, physical therapists, occupational therapists and nurses all work on this goal with the survivor.

The social worker on the team stays in touch with the family to see what kind of a support system the survivor has and updates the family on the survivor's progress. Where possible, families and stroke survivors also meet regularly with the stroke team.

Lourdes Regional Rehabilitation Center, for example, sees the family as an essential part of the rehabilitation treatment plan. Families act as consultants, giving the team important information about the stroke survivor's personality, goals and interests. They even attend therapy sessions so that they can begin to learn how to assist the survivor after he returns home.

Attending therapy sessions will teach the family how to help the stroke survivor.

Clearly, rehabilitation keeps each survivor on a demanding schedule of therapies as he works intensively toward specific goals. Let's take a closer look at what each member of the team works on.

Physical and Occupational Therapy: Moving toward Independence

Physical and occupational therapy form the backbone of the program to get a stroke survivor up, moving and back to performing the tasks of daily living. Physical therapists devise the survivor's exercise program and work on improving strength, coordination and basic movements. Occupational therapists work on helping survivors use their renewed strength and coordination to do specific activities like going to the bathroom, dressing, washing, shaving and eating.

Both physical and occupational therapists work on helping the survivor learn how to transfer from bed to chair, from wheelchair to toilet, from wheelchair to car, and from car to the rest of the world. Which "transfers" each therapist works on depends on the rehabilitation center, according to Joanna Beurgin, a registered physical therapist who is physical therapy supervisor at Lourdes Regional Rehabilitation Center. In fact, both kinds of therapists constantly complement each others' work—another reason the stroke team approach helps keep their activities coordinated.

Helen, a stroke survivor who had been living with her son before her stroke, entered Lourdes with a weakened hand grasp and a lot of balancing problems—she couldn't hold herself up even on the parallel bars in the physical therapy department used to help people learn to walk again. (Parallel bars are two long bars parallel to each other at hip level. The stroke survivor stands between them and grips each bar with a hand as he walks along.) But Helen kept up her work on the bars until at last she could walk with a cane, using it to help her balance.

Helen wanted to be able to cook for her son again, so occupational therapists worked with her on relearning kitchen skills—like how to reach high cabinets and use utensils with a weakened hand grasp. She had access to a full-size kitchen at Lourdes, where she practiced removing items from high and low shelves in a refrigerator and cabinets, walking and carrying food and cooking items, and standing at a stove preparing a meal. The combined efforts of these two departments meant that Helen did go home to live with her son again—and she does all the cooking herself. She's also tossed away her cane.

Sharon, another stroke survivor, couldn't walk at all or dress herself when she entered

Occupational and physical therapists help the stroke survivor learn new skills.

One woman learned how to cook with a weakened hand grasp.

Another woman learned
how to do anything—
including dress herself—
with one hand.

Physical and
occupational therapists
teach the stroke survivor
how to counteract the
effects of stroke.

Therapists can teach the
stroke survivor how to
judge distances.

Lourdes. After six weeks at Lourdes and a year of outpatient therapy, she is able to walk and can dress herself, even though she hasn't regained the use of her arm. "She is completely trained to do things with one hand," says Sandra Capoccia, a registered occupational therapist who worked with Sharon on learning to dress again. Occupational therapists can teach people to use assistive devices such as buttonhooks to help fasten buttons, pick up clothes and arrange them in place.

Physical and occupational therapists are experts at dealing with the varied effects of stroke. Depending on the survivor, they may be called upon to help with not only walking, using a wheelchair and balancing, but also with coordination problems, the loss of sensation in a paralyzed part of their body, difficulties in following directions, and difficulties understanding or speaking because of language impairments.

Other survivors suffer from *motor apraxia*, which means a stroke survivor may want to perform an activity and may have the muscular ability and coordination to do so, but he can't signal his muscles to do what he wants because the stroke has injured his brain.

Curiously, the survivor may be able to stand spontaneously, for example, but when asked to do it, he can't. In this case, therapists often assist the survivor in starting the task, which may then enable him to complete it himself.

But even if a stroke survivor can voluntarily perform a task—say, putting a coffee cup on the table—his or her perceptual skills may be damaged so that he can't judge distances correctly. He could miss the table and the cup would land on the floor. Or he could step off a curb and fall in the street. Or maybe he would bump into objects. Such problems with perception can cause safety problems, so therapists try to teach survivors to watch and compensate for errors in judgment.

In addition, many stroke survivors suffer from vision problems that keep them from seeing the side of their bodies affected by the stroke. And this impairment is often exacerbated by another problem: Some survivors forget that the paralyzed half of their bodies exists. This can be a great detriment to learning independent living skills.

Physical and occupational therapists help survivors overcome these problems as they are learning other skills. If a survivor who cannot see or has lost his sense of his paralyzed left side is eating, for example, a therapist can remind him to look toward the left side of the plate until eventually he learns to do this automatically.

A simple suggestion can make all the difference.

Tom, another stroke survivor at Lourdes Regional Rehabilitation Center, was unable to remember that his left side even existed because of the damage done by his stroke. He'd comb the hair only on the right side of his head. Putting on his glasses, he'd forget to unfold the left side of the glasses and they'd fall off his face. He'd eat only the food on the right side of his plate. And there were safety problems. Because he'd forget his left arm existed, he'd get it caught in the spokes of his wheelchair.

One man forgot his left side even existed.

Occupational therapists taught him to be much more aware of his left side by reminding him and practicing tasks over and over. Now he eats everything on his plate, combs his whole head and is in general much more aware of his left arm as being a part of his body, say his therapists at Lourdes.

Therapists helped him rediscover half of the world.

Whether a stroke survivor is eating, moving around, bathing or doing any other task, there are countless devices that can assist him or her to do the task more efficiently. Physical and occupational therapists help stroke survivors and their families use these devices and they can also be helpful in locating ones to rent or buy when a survivor returns home.

Among the most common equipment used by survivors are wheelchairs, walkers or canes, arm slings or arm trays to support a weak arm, hand splints, and leg braces to keep ankles and feet properly positioned. And there are countless small items to assist survivors with eating, grooming, dressing, bathing, playing or anything else.

After a stroke survivor returns home, many continue physical and occupational therapy, working both with therapists as outpatients and with family members. Their programs may include exercise, practicing the activities of daily living, and other therapeutic tasks. We'll talk more in chapter 12 about home therapy programs.

Rehabilitation doesn't stop when the stroke survivor returns home.

Speech/Language Therapy: to Talk, to Listen, to Understand

William, a stroke survivor, sat quietly in Tammy Feuer's office for his speech therapy session. Feuer, who is director of speech and hearing services at Lourdes Regional Rehabilitation Center, had just asked him to name the item she was showing him on a card. It was a picture of a towel.

As he concentrated fiercely, you could see William searching his mind for the word to go with a picture of something he so obviously recognized. He couldn't say the word, but he knew what to do with it. "You take a bath and dry off with it," he explained, partly through gestures. Later, when looking at a picture of a drum, he gestured like a drummer and this time, the word came. "You bang on a drum," he said.

There's more than one way to communicate.

Communication—that combination of speech, listening, reading, writing and gestures—is the one system, in the words of noted speech pathologist Martha Taylor Sarno, M.D.hc, associate professor of clinical rehabilitation medicine, "that is so uniquely human." When it is scrambled by a stroke, a condition called aphasia, no other disability leaves the stroke survivor feeling more cut off. More alone.

Aphasia scrambles communication.

"Imagine the aphasic stroke survivor who cannot talk properly, may not be able to understand the spoken word, read, write, gesture, handle numbers or money, tell the time, understand the calendar . . . recognize shapes, colors, etc.," says Norma Horwitch, a speech pathologist who is also the founder and director of the New Haven, Connecticut, Volunteer Stroke Rehabilitation Program, a unique group of volunteers who visit aphasics and help them practice communication skills.

"Imagine losing the ability to concentrate, be alert or aware, respond to stimuli where one thing leads to another, to handle the abstract . . . Communication is the great divide that separates us from animals and is the essence of our innate human behavior."

Communication is the essence of our humanity, says one speech pathologist.

Stroke survivor Marion Rasmussen, the articulate editor of a well-known newsletter for stroke survivors, recounts a harrowing tale of what she went through to regain her speech and language skills. "Learning to walk again made me feel elated, but it was nothing compared to making gains in understanding and communicating with others!

"At the beginning, I didn't even know my name," she says. "But if someone showed it to me, I could recognize it. I could see the beginning of words, but not the whole words. I could see letters in my mind, but not say them. To make the effort to form letters on paper, I had to practice all day long.

"I remember, in the hospital, I wanted a tossed salad so badly. I was trying to convey that to my speech therapist but she couldn't understand me. It was so frustrating. Finally, she figured out it was food I wanted. And from there she was able to figure out salad. She wrote it down and I practiced copying it so I could fill it out on the hospital menus."

Stroke survivors with speech difficulties feel that they are trapped in their brain.

Frustration. Humiliation. Alienation. These are just a few of the words aphasics who have recovered enough to say them tell us about their weary struggle to communicate effectively. Trapped inside a brain which is still intelligent, still functioning, they can no longer adequately say what they feel. Or, they cannot comprehend what others are saying to them. And, in some cases, they can't read or write or even recognize objects in pictures—so they may not be able to use those communication mediums to aid themselves either.

Friends and relatives should keep trying to communicate with the stroke survivor.

Cut off from a world that is so highly verbal, it's easy for aphasics to soon be isolated to an intolerable degree. Because they can be so difficult to understand, or have such difficulty understanding others, friends and relatives feel uncomfortable around them. So they stop visiting or trying to communicate with the aphasic. And then the one opportunity to practice communication skills that could help them regain some fluency with the nonaphasic world is gone.

Helping an aphasic learn to handle language again is obviously one of most crucial parts of rehabilitation. But it can also be one of the most difficult and challenging tasks. "The way we use language is so intensely personal, it differs for each one of us," says Dr. Sarno, who is director of speech-language pathology at the Howard A. Rusk Institute of Rehabilitation Medicine, New York University School of Medicine. "It's not like walking, which everybody does basically the same way." And there are no "crutches" to get you over the rough spots.

There are no "crutches" to get a stroke survivor with aphasia over the rough spots.

An additional frustration is that many aphasics may recover enough to communicate effectively, but still have residual problems that others fail to recognize. Marion Rasmussen speaks fluently, but says she still has trouble understanding television because actors talk so quickly.

Some aphasics would communicate better if others would speak more slowly.

"I'm hopeless with directions, too," she says.

"I have to have someone write them out for me so I can read them step by step."

Others, like aphasic Elaine Argetsinger, a former speech pathologist, cannot contribute effectively to group conversations because "I can't get a word in edgewise. I'm trying to get words from the wrong side of my brain and I can't react fast enough. Someone always gets a word in sooner," she says. "It's so frustrating, because I was so verbal before my stroke."

When a stroke survivor shows evidence of some form of aphasia, a speech pathologist (sometimes called a speech therapist) goes to work as soon as possible to evaluate what areas the aphasic is having trouble with. Some survivors will be primarily affected with *expressive aphasia*, which means their primary problems will be in expressing themselves through speaking and writing.

Expressive aphasia means the stroke survivor primarily has trouble talking.

Stroke survivors with *receptive aphasia*, on the other hand, have just the opposite problems. They are more likely to be unable to understand the printed or spoken word.

A third group of aphasics will have nearly equal difficulty in speaking coherently, understanding speech, reading and writing. And in the worst cases, a person with this *global aphasia*, as it is called, may have a complete loss of all language skills, according to Dr. Sarno.

Receptive aphasia means the stroke survivor primarily has trouble understanding what is said to him.

When a person has aphasia, he may be affected only mildly, or moderately, or the problem can be much worse—from severe to complete loss, such as we just described, says Dr. Sarno.

But whatever the severity of the problem, it is critically important for friends and family of an aphasic to remember that he is not mentally ill. The inability to communicate is not necessarily a sign of mental incompetency. "Regardless of the severity of his language loss, the person with aphasia must be treated as a mature, intelligent individual," says Dr. Sarno.

The aphasic is not mentally ill; he has a language problem.

A speech pathologist can help you find ways to communicate.

Improving language skills will keep the aphasic from becoming isolated.

Speech pathologists help families of aphasics learn the best forms of alternative communication with the person. If an aphasic can't speak, for example, he can occasionally write enough to get his point across. Or, if writing and speaking are both a problem, a system of gestures could be established. Even someone with global aphasia may be able to communicate through a series of index cards containing symbols.

Speech pathologists also help the stroke survivor by teaching other therapists how to communicate with the aphasic. They do this so that other therapists and nurses can reinforce the aphasic's efforts at regaining speech and language skills—usually through give-and-take conversations with the aphasic during daily therapy sessions. This is yet another example of how the team approach to stroke rehabilitation is so effective. If a speech pathologist wants a survivor to practice speaking, for example, he would encourage the occupational and physical therapists to chat with the aphasic as much as possible.

Speech pathologists also work with family members so that they, too, can reinforce the gains being made by the aphasic. Aphasics need plenty of extra support when they leave the rehabilitation center so that they can go on improving their language skills and remain unisolated from a world that still does not understand their disability, says Dr. Sarno.

Although aphasia is the most serious of all the language difficulties faced by stroke survivors, there are other speech problems they encounter, too, sometimes along with aphasia. If the muscles that produce speech in a stroke survivor are weakened or paralyzed, a condition known as *dysarthria*, he may slur words or, in some cases, be unable to produce sounds at all. Or other survivors have a condition known as *verbal apraxia*. Like the motor apraxia we described in the physical therapy section, people with verbal apraxia have muscles that would allow them to produce sounds, but they seem to have forgotten how to use them to do so.

Because speech and language skills are so complex and individualized, the disorders we've talked about here don't begin to fully describe the many complex ways that aphasia, dysarthria and apraxia can affect an individual's ability to communicate. That's why it's so important that a speech pathologist evaluate stroke survivors to determine what speech and language problems they have—and what's causing them—before recommending and following through with a therapy program.

You have to figure out what the problems are before you can solve them.

A therapist might assess a stroke survivor with speech and language problems by checking all forms of language skills: listening, speaking, reading, writing and gesturing. He would also check to see how well a survivor could name objects, do arithmetic, draw, imitate the speech of others and other skills. Then the therapist would conduct practice sessions with the patient to help him regain lost skills.

A speech therapist can help the stroke survivor regain lost skills.

The naming exercise that William, the stroke survivor from the Lourdes Regional Rehabilitation Center, was doing is one kind of practice. Speech pathologist Tammy Feuer also read small paragraphs to William and then asked him questions about the facts in them to help improve his listening skills. She also asked him to match a word at the beginning of a column to the exact word like it in a list of four or five similar words next to it. If the first word was "hat," for example, William had to find "hat" among such words as "cat," "home" and "mat."

But just as there are a multitude of ways that communication problems affect individual stroke survivors, so there are just as many ways to help someone regain his ability to communicate, says Dr. Sarno. The techniques are limited only by the therapist's creativity. And the stroke survivor's willingness to accept them.

Speech techniques are limited only by the therapist's creativity.

Psychological Therapy: Dealing with Post-Stroke Depression and Other Emotional Issues

Kay remembers well her first feelings after she "awoke" from her stroke. "I was dazed, in a state of shock—this just was not happening to me. I refused to accept it." Then Kay went from thinking she was in a bad dream to thinking, "Well, I'm going to beat this—in three months I'll be good as new." But soon Kay realized to her horror that she had a long road ahead of her. And at the end of it she might still be in a wheelchair, unable to speak and cut off from many of her old friends.

"What's left for me?" she thought. "A life where I burden my family and feel like an outcast?"

Many stroke survivors feel like outcasts from society.

For an overwhelming number of stroke survivors, Kay's agonizing response to the calamity of having a stroke is a common occurrence. In fact, it is part of a common response to any major life change, including serious illness and the death of a close friend or relative. It's nothing less than grieving.

Ideally, once the process of grieving for the person who was, but never will be again, is complete, a stroke survivor moves on to another stage. He accepts the new self and decides to make the best of his remaining abilities.

Post-stroke depression can be caused by your body's physical and emotional response to the stroke.

But, unfortunately, a majority of stroke survivors don't automatically move on to that stage of acceptance. They remain stuck in a post-stroke depression caused by their disabilities. Or, in some cases, they suffer from a kind of depression that is caused as much by their physical brain injuries as well as their situation.

Whatever the cause of the depression, however, the implications for stroke survivors are tragic. Some actually develop a kind of "pseudo-dementia" caused by the depression. In effect, the depression causes them to feel that they are losing their minds. Others don't make the gains in occupational, physical and speech therapy that they might have if they had not been depressed. In either case, their lives after the stroke are severely diminished. Needlessly.

Perhaps the most tragic fact of all is that most doctors don't realize that post-stroke depression is, in most cases, easy to identify and treat, according to the University of Maryland's Thomas R. Price, M.D., a leading researcher on the subject of post-stroke depression and director of stroke services at the university's medical school.

"I've wondered for a long time why post-stroke depression is so often missed by doctors. And I've come to feel that they are so overwhelmed by all the physical complaints a stroke survivor has that have to be attended to—the joints freezing, the bedsores, the heart disease, the speech problems. With all that, the doctor isn't thinking that perhaps the survivor's problems may be worse because of depression."

Post-stroke depression is often missed by doctors.

How common is post-stroke depression? Dr. Price and other researchers who have studied it say that more than *half* of all stroke survivors may be dogged by depression following a stroke. And in most survivors, the depression lasts for more than a year. The researchers have also discovered that when the depression is recognized and treated, the treatment is usually effective. And that's true whether the depression is caused by the survivor's reaction to his disabilities or if it's caused by brain injury.

More than half of all stroke survivors are clinically depressed.

"Families should *always* think of the possibility of depression in a stroke patient," believes Dr. Price. And that's especially important because your doctor may not. But even the survivor himself may not recognize the physical and mental symptoms because he's thinking that it's natural— "I'm feeling this way because of the stroke." So how do you tell if a stroke survivor is depressed?

Look for a lack of energy and a feeling of being easily fatigued, suggests Dr. Price. And also

A lack of energy and a loss of appetite may indicate depression.

watch out for a loss of appetite or weight, sleeplessness, pain that can't be traced to a cause, anxiety, irritability and gastrointestinal complaints like diarrhea or constipation.

Typical mental symptoms include an inability to make decisions, a lack of interest in other people or in the rehabilitation program, a sense of pessimism (especially about the future), a loss of self-esteem, loneliness, fear and an anger that the stroke survivor directs at himself.

Give your stroke survivor a short quiz and send the results to his doctor.

How can families convince doctors to explore the possibility of treating a stroke survivor for depression? Give them the results of a simple questionnaire for depression that Dr. Price and his colleagues use. (See the box, "Are You Depressed by Your Stroke?" on page 216.) When the results of the questionnaire—called the Center for Epidemiologic Studies Depression Scale (CES-D Scale)—were compared to more extensive testing, says Dr. Price, it identified three-quarters of the stroke survivors who were actually depressed. It's easy for nearly anyone to administer, but if you feel uncomfortable, ask a nurse to do it. Or ask the stroke survivor himself if reading and writing are not a problem.

In one study, antidepressant drugs helped stroke survivors progress further in rehabilitation than untreated survivors.

If a stroke survivor tests positive for depression, there are several ways to treat him. Antidepressant drugs, for example, have been shown to be very effective, says Dr. Price. In a study which compared depressed stroke survivors who took them with other similarly depressed survivors who had not, the pseudo-dementia of the treated survivors seemed to lift. And they made more progress in rehabilitation than the untreated survivors.

But even though most survivors can tolerate the drugs, they must be administered carefully since some antidepressants have side effects like sleepiness which could be counterproductive to a survivor's recovery. A psychiatrist can carefully monitor the survivor, however, and change the drug or the dosage if necessary, says Dr. Price.

Many stroke survivors are treated with psychotherapy, which can also be effective in helping stroke survivors out of their depressions. Jim Meier, a stroke survivor, says psychotherapy helped him "crawl out of the hole of depression" he found himself in after his stroke. "I found ways of seeing things more positively and knowing what my limitations were."

Meier advised his fellow survivors, in an article which appeared in the *Stroke Connection*, a newsletter written for and by stroke survivors, to talk to a doctor if they're feeling anxious or depressed. "Maybe you can't eliminate physical or mental difficulties, but talk does help you to understand and learn how to cope with them better. Speaking as a survivor, I assure you that psychotherapy works, and if it's needed, you should use it."

Psychotherapy can help stroke survivors understand what's happened and cope with it.

Many rehabilitation experts say that survivors and their families shouldn't underestimate the effect that a good rehabilitation program can have on some post-stroke depression. Because the emphasis is on activity, progress and improvement, it often helps the survivor's outlook. Just getting your bowels and bladder under control, or learning how to use a wheelchair to become independent again gives many survivors the boost they need to look at the future with renewed hope.

A rehab program that emphasizes activity, progress and improvement can also affect post-stroke depression.

Although post-stroke depression is the most obvious emotional challenge for the stroke survivor, there are other emotional changes to deal with. Many survivors suffer from a condition brought on by the brain injury called "emotional lability," in which they laugh or cry inappropriately. They also find it hard to control these extreme reactions.

"The more I'd try to control and stop it, the worse I'd get," said Jerry Bigoness, recalling the tears he said were so common in the months following his stroke. Jerry was part of a roundtable of

Emotional lability—inappropriate laughing or crying—is common after a stroke.

(continued on page 218)

Are You Depressed by Your Stroke? Take This Test and Find Out

Post-stroke depression. It's an incredibly common occurrence that experts say can prevent stroke survivors from making the rehabilitation gains they should. In some cases, it can cause a kind of "pseudo-dementia" that makes survivors feel like they're losing their minds.

The condition is usually treatable with drugs and/or psychotherapy, and the treatment is very effective, according to Thomas R. Price, M.D., of the University of Maryland. The trouble is, many doctors may not recognize post-stroke depression. Or they overlook it. So it may be up to stroke survivors and their families to call doctors' attention to it.

One piece of evidence that could help convince a doctor that the problem exists is a brief quiz, called the Center for Epidemiologic Studies Depression Scale (CES-D Scale). It can be administered by anyone—a family member or a nurse— yet it has the reliability of more formal testing often performed by psychiatrists, according to a study done by Dr. Price and other researchers.

We reprint the test here, with the scoring instructions below.

The Center for Epidemiologic Studies Depression Scale

Read or listen to each statement. Then pick from among the four numbers below the one that best describes how you felt or behaved in relation to that statement during the past week. The numbers correspond with the number of days during the week when you felt or acted that way.

0—rarely or none of the time (less than one day this week)

1—some or little of the time (one to two days this week)

2—occasionally or a moderate amount of time (three to four days this week)

3—most or all of the time (five to seven days this week)

1. I was bothered by things that usually don't bother me.
2. I did not feel like eating; my appetite was poor.
3. I felt that I could not shake off the blues even with help from my family or friends.
4. I felt that I was just as good as other people.
5. I had trouble keeping my mind on what I was doing.
6. I felt depressed (blue or down).
7. I felt that everything I did was an effort.
8. I felt hopeful about the future.
9. I thought my life had been a failure.
10. I felt fearful.
11. My sleep was restless.
12. I was happy.
13. I talked less than usual.
14. I felt lonely.
15. People were unfriendly.
16. I enjoyed life.
17. I had crying spells.
18. I felt sad.
19. I felt that people disliked me.
20. I could not get "going."

Scoring: Before adding up your score, reverse he numerical values on questions 4, 8, 12 and 16. These four are positive statements and therefore need to be valued differently for scoring. In other words, for those four questions, if you chose 3, give yourself a 0; 2, give yourself a 1; 1, give yourself a 2; 0, give yourself a 3.

(continued)

Are You Depressed by Your Stroke? Take This Test and Find Out—Continued

After you've done that, add up the numbers on all the questions. Dr. Price's study found that if the total number is under 16, you're probably not depressed. There are a few exceptions, however, so unless your score is under 4, you may want to discuss the possibility of post-stroke depression with your doctor.

---

stroke survivors, who were interviewed for this book at Courage Center, a doctor-based rehabilitation facility in Golden Valley, Minnesota. They told us that emotional lability was extremely common among all of them.

"That loss of control over your emotions is an awkward feeling," agreed Mary Balfour, another stroke survivor at the roundtable who suffered from lability. "You feel as though you have to explain what's happening," added Mel Smith, another survivor.

The survivors agreed that being in church or listening to music seemed to particularly bring on uncontrollable tears. "Any situation that's fairly emotional already—weddings, funerals, the kids being home at Christmas, saying grace—is also very difficult if you suffer from lability," said Smith.

On the bright side, the roundtable of survivors seemed to agree almost unanimously that emotional lability improves dramatically over time.

Lability improves dramatically over time.

But besides lability, stroke survivors can also experience real personality changes—a shy survivor can become uninhibited, a quiet one can become loud. And some lose a sense of social judgement or become extremely impulsive in other ways. These are also effects due to the brain injury.

Another emotional topic of real concern after a stroke is sexuality. It's a much-neglected area, agreed the members of our roundtable. And many said that doctors and nurses never broached the subject. "In the six years since my stroke, no one has ever talked to me about it," said one survivor.

Yet coping with changes in sexual relationships can be a very real anxiety. "I felt so paranoid after my stroke," said one survivor. "How could my husband still be interested in me? He had to move my paralyzed arm out of the way in bed. It was awful. I was sure he had to be having affairs."

"Doctors should tell you to expect sex to be different, so you don't feel like you're going nuts," said another stroke survivor. Another jokingly adds, "My wife was afraid she'd kill me!"

Sex is different—but it's still sex.

Why are the sexual concerns of stroke survivors so frequently ignored? Chris Papadopoulos, M.D., chief of cardiology at South Baltimore General Hospital, believes that there is still a myth that older people are no longer interested in sex. Yet half of all stroke survivors in one study resume sexual intercourse within six months.

Half of all stroke survivors resume sexual intercourse within six months, one study reports.

But while stroke survivors are definitely interested, they also have a lot of questions. And some problems. Many survivors find that depression, for example, interferes with their ability to have satisfying sex lives. Others have a negative self-image. Or they and their spouses may be afraid they'll cause another stroke. Yet if depression is treated and survivors are reassured that sexual activity is not more likely to cause a stroke than any other activity, often the problem is solved.

Some medications—especially those prescribed to control blood pressure or depression—can cause impotence in men, however, so it's a good idea to check with your doctor if you're having difficulties and you're on medication. Often the medication can be changed or adjusted to solve your problem.

Drugs that cause impotence can be changed or adjusted.

If a stroke survivor or spouse is having difficulty accepting himself or some of the role changes in his relationship (such as the wife becoming the breadwinner or the husband becoming the cook), or any other problems that interfere with a good sex life, don't hesitate to seek out a therapist experienced in sex counseling. Your doctor or therapist at the rehabilitation center should be able to recommend someone who can help.

The Social Worker: Helping Survivors and Families Face Post-Stroke Realities

When Evelyn and her husband and daughter arrived at the Lourdes Regional Rehabilitation Center where she was to undergo a stroke rehabilitation program, one of the first people they met with was Richard Heller, a social worker and part of the stroke rehab team who would be working with Evelyn. Heller sat down with the survivor and her family and listened as Evelyn's husband and daughter explained that they hoped Evelyn would be able to return home and that they would do everything they could to learn what they would need to do to care for her.

As Evelyn was evaluated by members of the stroke team, Heller kept her family updated on the team's goals for her and how she was making progress. He scheduled them in for appointments to learn how they could help Evelyn perform her physical exercises and transfer from her wheelchair to the bed. He also spent time with Evelyn and tried to help her explore her feelings about the stroke, but he came to feel that she might also need the help of the team's psychologist, so he referred her to him, as well.

As the time drew near for Evelyn to be discharged, Heller contacted the center's discharge planning department so the family could be referred to home health care services to help them

A social worker links family, rehab team and stroke survivor together.

with her home care. Both her husband and daughter were working full time, so they needed to hire a home worker who could give Evelyn the assistance she needed in dressing, getting to the toilet and eating. Evelyn was also going to continue with physical therapy at Lourdes and Heller helped them arrange transportation services to her therapy sessions.

He also looked over Evelyn's insurance policies to help find which benefits might be available for payment of the services needed for Evelyn. When it looked as if the insurance would not cover much of her care, he recommended resources in the community, like the local agency on aging that might be able to help with low-cost services.

"Evelyn" and her family are actually a composite of several families Heller has worked with at Lourdes. We've used them to illustrate the pivotal role played by a social worker in a stroke rehab program. The social worker not only offers emotional support to the survivor and family, he also keeps the stroke team informed of the survivor's family situation so it can tailor its rehabilitation efforts to suit the survivor's future needs. He offers practical help as the family faces the decisions involved in deciding how to care for their stroke survivor after he comes home.

"I also help the family to have realistic expectations about the stroke survivor's outlook," says Heller. "Are they fully aware of her deficits and what it will take to help her when she returns home? I try to be up-front and honest—I don't want to mislead them."

A social worker helps families and survivors look at one another realistically.

Recreation Therapy: Not Just for Fun

Many rehabilitation centers also use the services of recreational therapists and vocational counselors to help stroke survivors explore how they will use

Recreational therapists and vocational counselors can help the stroke survivor plan how to fill his days.

their time after returning home. For younger stroke survivors, returning to work may be an option. Older, retired survivors may want to explore new ways of taking part in recreational activities. Both younger and older survivors who are not returning to the paid work force may want to explore the creative opportunities to do volunteer work.

In chapter 10, we'll explore more fully all the various vocational, volunteer, and recreational opportunities and options a stroke survivor has once he returns home after a stay at a rehabilitation center. But for now, we'll talk specifically about the real contribution a recreational therapist makes to the stroke team and what a difference recreation can make during a stroke survivor's stay in a rehabilitation center.

"When you think about the money that is spent in this country on recreation and leisure time activities, it makes you realize how important recreational activities are in people's lives," says Dennis Dugan, a certified recreational therapist at Lourdes Regional Rehabilitation Center. "I try to find out what stroke survivors liked to do before their strokes, then I help them find ways to do those activities by adapting them when it's necessary."

Recreation isn't just for fun; it's also for fine-tuning many skills.

Dugan says that besides helping survivors think creatively about how they can continue to pursue the leisure activities they love, many recreational activities are therapeutic. Board games and playing cards, for example, can help survivors fine-tune their memories and other thinking skills, which may have been affected by their strokes. And physical activities—like the volleyball game he recently organized using a heavy balloon as the "ball"—help survivors increase their physical endurance while they have fun. "You can really get motivated if you're having fun," Dugan says.

Having fun is also a form of emotional therapy, he believes, especially for survivors overwhelmed by all that has happened to them. "It can help them get back into socializing, which many survivors need practice with if they're feeling bad about themselves or the way they look," Dugan says.

Recreation pulls stroke survivors back into society.

Rehabilitation Nursing: Offering a Helping Hand

Although we've talked about rehabilitation nurses throughout and how they reinforce all the different therapies the stroke survivor is practicing, they deserve a separate mention for the overall, continuous care they provide to stroke survivors during a stay at a rehabilitation center.

Nurses not only monitor a survivor's medical condition, administer medication and help him learn new skills, they also provide real emotional support and education to stroke survivors and their families. Nurses help families learn how to take care of a stroke survivor at home by giving them supervised opportunities to "practice" while he is still at the rehabilitation center.

Rehab nurses can teach caregivers how to help the stroke survivor at home.

They also provide the kind of reassuring support and encouragement many survivors need to reestablish good bowel and bladder habits. Achieving bowel and bladder control is one of the most important successes stroke survivors strive toward.

Putting It All Together

Reassurance. Support. Encouragement. They're the things so many survivors need to move successfully through rehabilitation and on to the rest of their lives. And some of the best people to give that support are other stroke survivors. Perhaps that's why so many survivors speak glowingly about the stroke clubs they join in communities all over the country. There, stroke survivors get together and share their joys and sorrows, successes

Stroke clubs are the foundation of regeneration.

A Day in the Life of a Stroke Survivor: The Rehabilitation Center Experience

Here's what a typical day might be like for a stroke survivor at a large rehabilitation center, according to Michele Miller, director of rehabilitation nursing at Lourdes Regional Rehabilitation Center, Camden, New Jersey.

7:30 A.M. John wakes up to see his cheerful nurse smiling down at him. And in no time at all he is practicing his morning ablutions, using the one-handed techniques he is learning from his occupational therapist. The nurse remains on hand to offer help and encouragement as John dresses and practices transferring from bed to wheelchair to toilet.

8:30 A.M. By this time, John has joined his fellow survivors for breakfast in the central dining room. "We like to encourage socialization—it helps patients deal with depression. And camaraderie makes them realize that they're not alone—others are going through the same thing," says Miller.

9:30 A.M. John begins his therapy in the physical therapy department, where he is starting to practice walking with the help of a leg brace.

10:30 A.M. John is off to occupational therapy, where he works on one-handed dressing techniques.

11:30 A.M. Speech therapy is next. Today, the therapist is working with John on his listening skills. He reads a brief story to him and then questions him on the details he remembers.

12:00 M. Lunch, again with fellow rehabilitation participants.

and failures, ups and downs. They also learn what's important in rehabilitation. And in life.

As stroke survivor Walt Collins says, "I have also learned to love myself. The old Walt Collins is

"We have been given a second chance at life."

1:00 P.M. John takes a well-deserved nap before starting his afternoon therapy sessions. "We try to schedule in one rest period sometime during the therapy day or before dinner," says Miller. "Of course, at the beginning, stroke survivors may need more than that—but we generally try to discourage too much lying in bed. The more you stay in bed, the weaker you get."

2:30 P.M. John is back in the physical therapy department doing range-of-motion exercises and practicing the operation of his wheelchair.

3:30 P.M. Occupational therapy again, where he is practicing kitchen skills in a kitchen set up there.

4:30 P.M. John spends some time with a social worker. They discuss the many ways to cope with the depression he is feeling.

6:00 P.M. Dinner with the other patients.

7:00 P.M. The weekly in-house stroke club meeting is tonight. Each of the survivors shares the progress he has made during the past week. It's hard for John, who has difficulty speaking, to explain his progress. But the group gives him the time to speak. And with the help of Lourdes staffers who are acquainted with his case, he is able to update the group on his gains. On nights when the stroke club does not meet, John spends time in recreation therapy—playing games, socializing and relaxing.

8:30 P.M. John is back in his room, where his nurse helps him to shower. Since his therapy sessions begin early the next day, there won't be the time in the morning.

10:00 P.M. John calls it a night.

gone and I love the new me. Remember one thing, stroke survivors: We have been given a second chance at life. There have been many who never had it."

Chapter 10

Going Home: Preparing Yourself

J ean sat down for the first time since Bill's stroke six weeks before and contemplated the road ahead of her. Her feelings ran the gamut, from relief that her husband had survived the stroke and was making gains in rehabilitation to sheer panic at all the millions of details she had to take care of before he could come home—the ramp that needed building, the bathroom that had to be converted to accommodate a disabled person, the special clothes and equipment she wanted to get for Bill to make his life more independent and the home health aide she would need to hire, at least for a while, to help Bill while she worked at her part-time job. And how in the world was she going to pay for all this? It looked like their insurance policies covered very little after Bill left the rehabilitation center.

Jean hadn't even had time to think about what Bill was going to do to fill his days now that it looked as though he would retire from his job. Of course there would probably be some outpa-

The caregiver's life.

tient therapy sessions at first—another thing she needed to arrange. But what about the rest of the time? And what about the time when those therapy sessions ended? Bill had some fairly serious speech problems and Jean could see already how difficult it was for his own children to communicate with him. How would they maintain their relationship with him? How would their friends? Would they just stop visiting?

What about you?

Finally, down at the bottom of that long list of concerns, Jean spared about a minute and a half to think about herself. She had spent 23 years caring for her children and putting their needs first. Now would she spend the rest of her life putting Bill's needs ahead of her own? Would she ever have the time to do some of the things she had planned when the children grew up? And what about the plans for the future she and Bill had dreamed about? Would they ever materialize now?

Jean is not a real person. She's a composite of all of us who care for stroke survivors, all of us who begin life after stroke in a whirlwind of detail.

After a stroke, life begins as a whirlwind of detail.

But as overwhelming as those first weeks preparing for the homecoming may seem, it's really afterward that many caregivers face the full force of what lies ahead. And at that moment—when both caregivers and survivors need support the most—the rug is often pulled out from under them. Insurance payments for continuing therapy run out. Friends stop dropping by. Everyone gets on with his own life. But for the caregivers and stroke survivors, a new life is just beginning, one for which they had very little time to prepare. One for which they have received scant training.

That's why this chapter is for you—the spouses, children, siblings and close friends of stroke survivors. Consider this—and all the succeeding chapters—your guide to ideas, extra hands and spiritual strength.

There is help.

So let's talk for a few minutes about you, the caregiver who's in charge of this enormous task.

It's the Family That Has the Stroke

"Caregivers need care, too!" says Jane Royse, one of this country's most ardent spokespersons for the needs of caregivers.

But because the focus is so much on the survivor, the caregiver's needs are often woefully unmet. "I wish just once someone would first ask me how *I* am," a caregiver told Royse, who conducts caregiver support groups for the Wilder Foundation, a social services agency in St. Paul. "Nobody calls me by my name anymore, "I'm 'John's wife' to everyone," complained another. And a third caregiver told Royse, "If you see the two of us, I'm the tired, drawn-out one with my hair mussed. He's all clean and showered and rested—he looks great."

You can tell who's the caregiver by how he or she looks—tired, drawn-out and mussed.

Clearly these caregivers—and their children—are hurting, says Royse. And in some cases they're grieving because they feel they've lost that person in their lives on whom they could always depend.

Everyone in the family grieves for the friend who is "lost."

It's because of these kinds of problems that experts who counsel the families of stroke survivors say the entire family really has a stroke, not just the stroke survivor. And, like the stroke survivor, family members go through periods of denial, anger, depression and acceptance. It's just that many caregivers don't give themselves permission to have any negative feelings—they feel guilty or uncomfortable about them.

Learn How to Handle Your Anger

"But negative feelings are normal in a situation like yours," says Royse to the families of stroke survivors. "There's a fine line between love and hate. And, yes, you *can* feel both. Think about the anger you may be feeling toward the survivor and try to separate the person from the sickness. Would you still be angry with him if he weren't

Anger, depression and other uncomfortable feelings are normal.

sick? If you would not, you know it's the sickness that's causing your anger—not the person.

"I encourage caregivers to get help in learning how to channel those angry feelings and deal with them in appropriate ways," says Royse.

If the survivor you're caring for is treating you badly—foisting his or her anger off on you, for example—try to tell yourself that it's not your husband (or wife) who is treating you that way, it's the stroke. "It helps if you can look at the stroke as the place to put all the blame," Royse suggests. "Tell yourself, 'if he could help it, he wouldn't be that way to me.' "

Blame the stroke, not the person who had it.

"I can't say two sentences before my husband cuts me off and tells me he doesn't want to hear any more," says one stroke survivor's wife. "He belittles me and criticizes me—he's just a different person than he was before the stroke," she says. "But I've learned to accept it as a part of his stroke. And I think of what my son tells me: 'Mom, that isn't Dad anymore.' I've also learned how to detach myself. It doesn't mean I don't still love him or care about him, or that I would desert him. I just won't let myself be a part of his problem."

Anger and negative feelings can also surface, as spouse/caregivers cope with the loss of the husband-wife relationship they once had—one which is probably very changed after a stroke, says Royse. "The loss of that relationship often means no longer having your best friend, your companion, your lover—the person who shared your life," she wrote to one very troubled caregiver.

"He used to be very affectionate, thoughtful, humorous, and very considerate of me," writes one wife of a stroke survivor. "And I really miss those qualities in him now. No longer can he buy me a present, hold the door open for me, or give me a meaningful hug."

It's normal that those angry feelings can be directed toward others, says Royse—at other couples who haven't experienced a stroke, at family and friends, and at the stroke survivor, too. But you shouldn't have to cope with those feelings all alone, she says. Seeking help, through professional counseling, support groups and your church or synagogue is a good idea.

You're not expected to handle all the anger by yourself.

Take Care of Yourself

Besides dealing with negative feelings, Royse says, caregivers should not feel guilty about having their own needs. "Unless you take care of yourself, you won't be able to care for others over a long period of time," she says. Many caregivers, because of the overwhelming tasks they have confronting them, give up their social lives, their activities and time for themselves. Add all that sacrificing to the hard work and losses of caregivers and it can contribute to an unbearably high level of stress—unless the caregiver takes a break and insists on time for himself.

You can't take care of someone else's needs until your own are met.

"Don't sit in that house—get out and take some time for yourself," says Betty Anderson, whose husband, Joe, is a stroke survivor. "Joe used to tell me 'Go, or you're going to crack.' And I'd say to him—you're right. And if I crack—where does that leave you?"

But even if your stroke survivor doesn't push you to think about yourself, do it anyway, agree Royse and other caregivers. "My husband still doesn't tell me to go do something for myself. I have to take the initiative and just do it," says another caregiver.

"Caregivers shouldn't be expected to go beyond a normal amount of giving. They need to set limits and learn to say no without feeling guilty," says Royse. "If the person you're caring for wants a drink of water—don't necessarily rush off to get it. Encourage him to get the drink. Or if he wants a snack half an hour after you've finished lunch, tell

Learn your limits.

him you need to rest or finish what you're doing. You'll get the snack in another half hour."

Since many caregivers are women, points out Royse, they—in particular—need to learn to be assertive about their needs. And assertiveness is an attitude many women don't practice enough. "Women are expected to give and give and give and sacrifice ourselves while caring for someone else—even at the expense of our own health and well-being," she says.

But male caregivers have their own set of problems. "If I had it to do over again, I'd take some time for myself," says Skip Lee, referring to the first months and years after his wife, Marcia, had a stroke. "I felt like I was the one who was responsible. I was indispensable. I think I would have weathered it better emotionally if I'd just asked for help sometimes. But I was 'tough'—I thought I should be able to handle this myself."

Learn How to Ask for Help

Asking for help is probably the number one talent caregivers need to cultivate in themselves, according to all the caregivers we interviewed. "There are two good things that have come out of this," says Betty Anderson, referring to her husband's stroke. "One, I've learned patience—Lord, you have to. And two, I've learned to ask for help. I was proud and I didn't want to ask. But every time I did, I found others who were willing. And you have to ask—people don't know unless you tell them you need it. They're always willing—but you *have* to ask."

"We don't live in a society where people automatically help you," agrees Royse. "When a caregiver begins the job of caring for another person at home, it can be like a funeral. Everyone comes by, bringing casseroles and offering help—saying 'call me if you need anything.' But after two or three weeks, all those people go back to their

Then learn to ask for help.

In our society, people don't automatically extend a helping hand, says one woman.

lives. Then, it's up to the caregiver to take the initiative and ask for assistance."

And you have to be plain about your needs, says Royse. "I hear mothers who say 'my daughters won't help out.' Then I talk to the daughters and they tell me 'I asked Mom what help she needed but she couldn't tell me.'"

If you're having trouble asking for help, or if relatives don't seem to be responding to your requests, you might consider drawing up a written family agreement among them, suggests Joan Ellen Foyder in her excellent and practical book, *Family Caregiver's Guide*. Foyder's book contains copies of such an agreement, in which family members specify what help they can offer shopping, providing transportation or relieving the caregiver a specified number of times per month. When such an agreement is in writing, Foyder reports, family members will tend to be realistic about the help they can actually provide. And the written reminder serves as a stimulus to make good on promises.

Prepare a written agreement specifying which family member does what and when.

Royse says that caregivers need to give themselves permission to ask for help, even if it makes them feel uncomfortable. "Caregivers often get stuck in the caregiving role. It's hard for them to consider other options. But there's usually another option. It may not be ideal and you may not be crazy about it, but sometimes we have to let go of some things to survive."

Look for Respite Care

If family members or friends are not available to relieve you occasionally from caregiving responsibilities, there are usually other sources of what is called "respite care" in the community, according to the National Council on Aging (NCOA). Volunteers and paid companions can come into your home on a regular or as-needed basis, adult day-care programs can provide your survivor with

Volunteers, paid companions and adult day care can give you a break.

(continued on page 240)

Community Stroke Aftercare Programs: Three Very Special Examples

Stroke survivors and their families are in desperate need of supportive services, especially in the months and years after the "acute" stroke emergency is over. Although buoyed up at first by rehabilitation programs and hospital services, survivors and their families often feel cast out to sea after these services end. But some communities have developed some very special lifelines to help them. Here's a look at three exceptionally caring programs. We provide contact names and addresses for all three programs, in case you, or someone in your community, would be interested in starting a group modeled after one of these.

Evergreen Stroke Association/ARISE

Although the Evergreen Stroke Association had its roots in one small, informal stroke club, it has grown into a unique program serving stroke survivors all over the Seattle, Washington, area. The association, which is a program of Family Services, an umbrella social services agency, receives funding from the United Way and other sources. It offers a wide array of innovative programs for families fortunate enough to live in that area.

The association provides stroke survivors and their families with social support and education. Volunteers, who are usually stroke survivors or their spouses, visit new survivors and their families in the hospital to offer reassurance and provide a packet of materials about coping with stroke. They see to it that survivors and their families know about the many stroke clubs throughout the area which are aligned with the association. And they lend books on stroke and rehabilitation.

The association also provides peer counseling (performed by stroke survivors and their spouses) and other professional counseling for those who need it to deal with the emotional aftermath of stroke. And Evergreen doesn't forget about caregivers' and other family members' needs. Support groups for them are available, too. Social opportunities also abound, because the association sponsors picnics, dinners, outings and tours, as well as a recreational camp.

But its services don't end there. The association provides meaningful volunteer opportunities for stroke survivors who, after receiving Evergreen services, often turn around and provide them for others. When support from other survivors has seen you through a black time after a stroke, it's easy to return the favor.

The association also acts as an advocate for stroke survivors in the community, raising consciousness and spreading the word about stroke prevention. During June, which the association has designated stroke awareness month, it sponsors public service announcements, hospital forums, seminars, brochures, health fairs and other media events.

And finally, the association operates ARISE, which is a two-year, post-rehabilitation day program for stroke survivors. The structured program helps build survivors' skills and confidence and provides a bridge back to the community. The association started ARISE when it became clear that most survivors needed more support and rehabilitation after their relatively brief rehabilitation center stays. But survivors either couldn't afford it or they couldn't find it.

ARISE participants meet three days a week and work on goals they've set in several areas, including physical and occupational therapy, speech therapy, cognitive and intellectual challenge, vocational/volunteer rehabilitation, and

(continued)

Community Stroke Aftercare Programs: Three Very Special Examples—Continued

recreational therapy. The social benefits of working on rehabilitation goals with a group of survivors who have a lot in common makes ARISE a very special, very effective program.

For survivors who cannot afford the relatively small fees which ARISE charges for its services, there's a sliding scale, so that no survivor who could benefit from the program needs to be turned away. Donations from the United Way and other fund-raising efforts cover extra costs for these survivors. The program also receives some insurance reimbursement, which many survivors can take advantage of.

To learn more about the Evergreen Stroke Association and its many programs, contact director Johanna Padie, Evergreen Stroke Association, 9423 Southeast Thirty-sixth Street, Mercer Island, WA 98040. You may want to plant an "evergreen in your community tomorrow.

OPUS: Organization of People Undaunted by Stroke or Other Disabilities

"One of the worst things you can do to stroke survivors is to do everything for them. It takes away their dignity," says Ruth Kamerman, volunteer director of a three-day-a-week day program for disabled adults called OPUS (Organization of People Undaunted by Stroke or Other Disabilities). So OPUS does just the opposite. It's an organization where stroke survivors (and other disabled people) do for themselves and others.

When the work of keeping their own organization going is done (everything from making and selling holiday wreaths to cleaning up the church hall where they meet), OPUS members spend much of the rest of their time doing charitable work for other volunteer organizations. (A typical activity might be stuffing envelopes for an organization and preparing them for mailing.) They do so many good works for others, in fact, that they were honored by their community as Volunteer Group of the Year.

"Stroke survivors' self-images are often decimated after they come home from the rehabilitation hospital. They've done nothing but take, take, take." says Kamerman. "We try to help them restore their dignity by giving to others for a change. That's the cornerstone of our organization."

And the giving doesn't end with volunteer work. Kamerman says the less-physically afflicted members of OPUS are constantly helping those with greater problems."They hang up each others' coats. They help open lunches. They help each other get to the bathroom," she says. "It's really a low-pressure, family atmosphere—very much unlike the structured and more demanding medical programs many of them have been through. They often find this more palatable."

Along with their other activities, OPUS members can take advantage of exercising with a physical therapist several days a week, playing games, doing crafts and just generally socializing with each other. "Many of the survivors who come here would never get out of the house otherwise," says Kamerman. Although she and the small band of volunteers who help out are not paid and the group gets no federal funding ("We don't want those forms to fill out."), they do get a small New York state legislative grant to help pay the costs of transporting OPUS members to the church hall where they meet. A specially equipped van picks members up from a wide area.

With that small grant and their fund-raising efforts, OPUS is easily able to manage its small annual budget of under $40,000, says Kamerman. Each day that they are there, OPUS members must contribute some money, but it can never be

(continued)

Community Stroke Aftercare Programs: Three Very Special Examples—Continued

more than $2 a day. "This fits in well with our philosophy of giving, not taking." OPUS members also contribute up to a dollar toward defraying the cost of having the physical therapist visit them twice a week. They bring their own lunches and most of the time they come by themselves, giving their families a much-needed, low-cost break from their caregiving duties.

"Often, stroke survivors become very narcissistic and self-consumed when they first begin to cope with their disabilities. But when they come here, they start to think more about each other and less about themselves. These folks really care about each other," says Kamerman.

For more information on OPUS, you can contact Ruth Kamerman, OPUS, Organization of People Undaunted by Stroke or Other Disabilities of Westchester County, 101 North Central Avenue, Hartsdale, NY 10530.

The Volunteer Stroke Rehabilitation Program (VSRP)

It was a serendipitous chance meeting on a train that got the Volunteer Stroke Rehabilitation Program (VSRP) on its feet. VSRP founder and director Norma Horwitch, who is a speech pathologist, was traveling from Boston to New Haven, when she realized that sitting close by was Patricia Neal, the actress who had suffered a series of massive strokes during the 1960s. She and Neal struck up a conversation and the two became friends.

Horwitch learned about the world of confusion, frustration, despair and boredom in which Neal lived when she lost her language skills—the condition known as aphasia. But Neal also told her about the unusual and loyal band of volunteers which her ex-husband, Roald Dahl, gathered around her as she recuperated from her strokes in England. These volunteers helped her read, practice speaking, handle money and do other tasks. With this day-in, day-out help, Neal recovered her language skills. One of the volunteers who worked with Neal, Valerie Eaton-Griffith, decided to expand the volunteer program to help other aphasics, and now England has close to 100 chapters of the Volunteer Stroke Scheme, founded by Eaton-Griffith.

Horwitch met Eaton-Griffith and the rest, as they say, is history. The New Haven speech pathologist, who had worked in a public school system for 16 years, decided to start the Volunteer Stroke Rehabilitation Program in her area. The idea behind it is a simple one. Aphasics need lots of help and practice to regain some of their lost language proficiency. But most people don't understand that, so they tend to shy away from speaking to the aphasic, who may be difficult to communicate with. He quickly loses contact with the world, as even family and close friends back away.

That's where VSRP volunteers come in. A number of different volunteers visit an aphasic each week, and each of them spends about an hour and a half with him or her at a time. They usually do an activity which helps the aphasic relax and communicate better. Volunteers don't need formal training, says Horwitch. "All that is required is a head, a heart, compassion, some orientation and the willingness to help a fellow human being."

Even when an aphasic is still involved in formal speech therapy, he can benefit from the complementing services provided by volunteers, says Horwitch. And even more important, when therapy stops (usually because insurance funding runs out), the volunteers are still there to help aphasics make further strides.

(continued)

Community Stroke Aftercare Programs: Three Very Special Examples—Continued

VSRP also operates aphasia clubs, which meet regularly so that aphasics can take advantage of more social stimulation. Currently, VSRP has four chapters in Connecticut and is trying to establish a program in New York City.

"The relationships that develop between these aphasic stroke survivors and their volunteers are very beautiful ones. Volunteers help aphasics keep boredom at bay," says Horwitch. And, they open the world up again for many grateful stroke survivors.

For more information on VSRP, contact Norma C. Horwitch, Volunteer Stroke Rehabilitation Program, Inc., 96 Westwood Road, New Haven, CT 06515.

some socializing time while you take a break and nursing homes can provide for short-term stays.

To find out where such care is available, check with your area agency on aging (check the yellow pages of your phone book under "Senior Citizens" or the blue pages under "Aging"), other caregivers, your church or synagogue, senior citizen centers and other community groups.

Some community groups may provide respite on a voluntary or sliding fee scale, so don't reject this idea because you're afraid you won't have enough money to pay for it. And, if you feel uncomfortable about leaving your survivor with a "stranger," talk about this concern with other caregivers who have used respite services, advises the NCOA. They may be able to address your concerns and answer your questions.

Senior centers, churches, synagogues and other community groups can help you find respite care.

Find Some Friends
in the Same Boat

Once you've begun to ask for help, look for things to do and ways to give yourself enjoyable—and therapeutic—breaks from your caregiving responsibilities. There are really two ways to go, say the caregivers we spoke with. One excellent option is to find a support group of other caregivers. "I *had* to talk to other people who understood what I was going through," says Judy, the wife of another stroke survivor. "My friends meant well, but they didn't understand."

And Val, another caregiver, adds, "Get involved with a group as soon as you can—it saved my sanity!"

A support group can save your sanity.

Caregiver support groups are an idea whose time has come, says Royse, who has been involved in such groups for nine years. There are at least 300 such groups around the country.

How can you find out if a support group exists in your area? Check first with the rehabilitation center or hospital where your stroke survivor stayed. They often sponsor such groups or may be able to refer you to one in the area. You can also check with your local agency on aging.

A local rehab center or hospital will know about stroke support groups.

If none of these leads works out, write or call NCOA's Caregivers of the Aging Program. (For NCOA's address, with information on how to join Family Caregivers of the Aging, see the appendix, "The Family Caregivers' Resource Guide.") This relatively new program was started solely to help family caregivers and it can help you find a support group in your area. If no group exists, the NCOA program can provide you with how-to materials to start your own.

The Family Caregivers of the Aging Program can also provide resources.

Another group that can help you find a caregivers' support group in your area is Children of Aging Parents (CAPS), a group that addresses not only the needs of children but also those of spouses who are caregivers. CAPS can also provide help and how-to materials for starting your own group. (See the appendix for address.)

You might want to contact your local rehabilitation facility to see if it would consider providing funds and space for starting a caregivers' group. They could also hire Royse—to provide initial training on how to organize and run the group. Write to her c/o The A.H. Wilder Foundation, 919 LaFond Avenue, Saint Paul, MN 55104.

A support group gives you a chance to discuss common problems, brainstorm about solutions and generally lend moral support for the tremendous job you are doing. But Royse says it should also be a place where you can go to talk about yourself. "I tell groups, 'this group is for you,' " she says. " 'So don't spend all your time talking about the stroke survivor, the disease or illness. Spend time talking about care for the caregiver.' "

A support group helps you brainstorm for solutions to common problems.

Talk about Anything but Strokes

Royse also suggests that caregivers spend some time every day speaking to someone about anything other than the survivor or the stroke. And she also advises caregivers to see old friends not connected to the stroke survivor. "Spend time talking about yourself, your grandchildren or even the weather. It's easy to think nothing is happening in the world but caregiving."

Talk about yourself every day.

One caregiver we interviewed who has a particularly difficult home caring situation spends several weeks at a time visiting friends and relatives in another city while her son takes over caregiving duties. "When I come back, I can cope with it all a little better again," she says.

Having other friends to share your own hopes and dreams can fill a critical gap you may be feeling if the stroke survivor isn't able to be the partner/parent/sibling/friend he once was. If your spouse was someone you depended on for a lot of emotional support, for example, and now he can no longer do that because of some of the effects of stroke, a close friend or relative can help you adjust to that change.

Sometimes the person doesn't have to be a grown-up either. "There's nothing more wonderful than my two little grandchildren telling me, 'Grandma, we love you,' " says one caregiving spouse. "I don't get that from my husband anymore."

Are there positive changes that caregivers report? Many spouses are proud of the skills they've learned that once were solely their partners' jobs. "I became the plumber and a lot of other things," laughs caregiver Betty Anderson. "But I also quickly learned that I couldn't do everything. After my back started giving me trouble, I hired someone to mow the lawn and shovel snow."

"I can put gas in my car, check the oil and transmission fluid and put air in my tires," says another caregiver proudly.

And caregivers were unanimous in recommending that you give up being a perfectionist about how your home looks. "I make priorities. I have left the beds unmade and the dishes dirty when they were low on the list," says Anderson. Adds another survivor, "I just do the necessary things—I wash clothes and vacuum when it looks like the rugs can't stand it anymore."

Give up being a perfectionist about your home.

A study of the caregivers of stroke survivors, performed by Brown University School of Medicine's Rebecca A. Silliman, M.D., Ph.D., and her colleagues, showed that caregivers generally report an increased sense of self-esteem at being able to manage their loved ones' illnesses.

Managing a stroke survivor's life will build your self-esteem.

Those same caregivers, however, reported more personal ill health—about twice that seen in their age groups in the general community.

Caregivers also worried about what would happen if they, the caregivers, could no longer provide care. And they felt some of the same stresses we've already mentioned like a diminished social life and the tremendous responsiblities of caring for the stroke survivor. Taking the time for social activities and getting help from family members can ease the stresses of caregivers, the study's authors concluded.

If your social life is suffering because your "couple" friends have stopped calling you to go out, Royse encourages you to take the initiative and call them. If your spouse cannot go out, feel comfortable going out on your own or with a friend.

"It's all right to join other people as a single," says Royse. "Many caregivers are in the unusual situation of being married, but leading a single life."

Your true friends will stick with you; the others don't count.

Caregivers say their contacts with old friends after the stroke really teach them who their friends are. Your friends stick with you, they say, acquaintances do not. But don't worry about the acquaintances, they advise. It's the friends who count.

What many caregivers, especially spouses, have the hardest time adjusting to is what they perceive as their diminished dreams for the future. Like the survivors, they too may have had plans that are unrealistic after the stroke.

"My husband and I loved camping and being out in nature," says one stroke caregiver. "We had a camping van and had planned to travel. But he can't drive anymore and I don't feel able to drive the van. He lost that dream, but I did, too." Caregivers need to talk through these feelings with counselors and support groups, and work toward a coming-to-terms with them.

Besides organized groups, there are also other supportive services for caregivers these days. All three of the organizations we talked about above produce newsletters and other printed materials of help to caregivers. The National Council on the Aging's Family Caregivers of the Aging program offers *Caregiving* newsletter, a publication full of useful tips and hints, which is mailed to members of the program. And the program produces two sets of pamphlets for caregivers on a wide range of practical issues.

Support group newsletters are loaded with tips on how to cope.

CAPS also produces two newsletters—*Advice for Adults with Aging Parents or Dependent Spouses* and *The CAPSule*—while Jane Royse and the Wilder Foundation have a pamphlet for caregivers filled with advice about how to take care of yourself.

Caregivers can also join the Courage Stroke Network, a nationwide network for stroke survivors and their families, based at the Courage Center in Golden Valley, Minneapolis. The group's newsletter, *Stroke Connection*, is one of the most helpful, practical and inspirational newsletters around for people going through the stroke experience. The newsletter is written and edited by stroke survivors and their caregivers, and the thought-provoking insights by these two groups provide you with a kind of "written" support group.

While grappling with the many emotional and life-altering changes going on in your life, you, the caregiver, must also be arranging for a million and one practical details in caring for a stroke survivor. This task shouldn't be another source of stress for you. So, to help you get organized so that things run smoothly, the next chapters will focus on the three main caregivers' tasks.

- Outfitting your home and buying or renting equipment that's especially needed for stroke survivors with disabilities
- Arranging home health and homemaker services

- Helping the survivor—and you—get on with your lives, through continuing rehabilitation therapy, recreational, social and work opportunities

Read on and relax. You can handle it all.

Chapter 11

Nuts and Bolts: Preparing Your Home

Adapting your home to make it easier and safer for a stroke survivor, as well as the caregiver, doesn't necessarily involve a lot of time and money. It all depends on the existing house and the individual disabilities the survivor is coping with, say the home modification experts we consulted. Many adaptations are easy to do yourself; others may require the services of a contractor or other expert in accessible home improvements.

You can do many of the necessary home modifications yourself.

But before you go all out with an expensive renovation, there's one basic question you need to ask, says Shannon McGurran of the Courage Center in Golden Valley, Minneapolis—especially after the period of formal rehabilitation. "Are permanent modifications necessary due to the extent of the disability—or will temporary modifications work until the individual has gained back increased independence through rehabilitation and will no longer require the use of modifications?"

Do you need a temporary or permanent modification?

A stroke survivor who is working toward walking again may not need the permanent entrance ramp you're thinking of building for his wheelchair, for example. A temporary one would do the trick. Or you may not need to redo the bathroom to accommodate a wheelchair. A portable, hand-held shower head, along with a small, inflatable pool, can be used in the kitchen where there is ample floor space.

If you are planning a ramp or other major structural changes in your home, you may find it difficult to locate a contractor who is experienced in remodeling for disabled people, says Ronald L. Mace, who heads the design firm Barrier Free Environments, Raleigh, N.C. Mace is an architect and a nationally known advocate of barrier-free design.

If you need a builder, have him consult with therapists at your rehab center.

McGurran agrees. "Many contractors would not know how to properly and safely build a ramp, for example, that is not too steep or provides safety features to avoid falling off," she says. Your best bet is to ask other stroke survivors or disabled people which contractors/designers they used and whether they were satisfied. Or, if you have no referrals, your builder could consult with the rehabilitation therapists at the center your survivor is using, says McGurran. They may be able to advise him on the correct width and slope for a ramp, for example.

Mace's firm acts as a consultant on building projects all over the United States. "We can review the plan your builder is proposing to see if he really is making your home accessible," he says. "Then we can suggest changes that will improve the design. Or we can do the original design for you and then oversee its execution by a local builder. We may also be able to refer you to a suitable design expert in your area, because we have contacts all over the country."

Barrier Free Environments will review your plans.

Barrier Free Environments publishes a wide array of guides and books on accessible housing. You can obtain a publication list from them. Finally, says Mace, the firm can simply answer by phone questions you may have on any aspect of accessible housing. (Mace can be reached at Barrier

Free Environments. The address is in the appendix, "The Family Caregivers' Resource Guide.")

Another source of printed information on accessible housing is the Paralyzed Veterans of America, which provides guides to different areas of the house, with illustrations and specifications which a home remodeler can follow. (See the appendix for the group's address.)

The best way to discuss home modifications, according to McGurran and Mace, is to go step-by-step through your house. At some point during your survivor's stay, a therapist from the rehabilitation center may do just that with you and advise you on potential problem areas. Here are a few common problem areas with some sample solutions suggested by McGurran and Mace.

Go step-by-step through your home to see what needs to be modified.

Entrances and exits. Getting in and out of the home can often be a major problem for a stroke survivor. Sturdy handrails and nonskid tape (for slippery steps) might be all that's needed if your survivor is walking and able to negotiate stairs. A ramp might be your first consideration if he is not. Consider a temporary ramp if it looks like the survivor may be in a wheelchair for only a limited period. This is also a good idea if you live in rented housing. You can buy a prefabricated ramp which can be disassembled if you move.

Check your entrances and exits.

If you're installing permanent access, wood ramps are the least expensive, but may have to be replaced periodically. If you build with wood, make sure there's space between the boards to allow melting ice to drip through in winter. Masonry and concrete ramps are more expensive than wood but will last longer. Ramps should always be built so that for every 1 inch of rise there are 12 inches in ramp length.

While you're conquering the steps problem, consider this: Can the wheelchair fit through doorways throughout your home? Most can, but if it can't, don't despair. Simply changing the standard hinges to clear swing hinges allows the door to swing all the way back behind the door frame and

Switching the hinges on your door can make all the difference.

out of the door opening, adding a critical 1½ to 2 inches to your entranceway. If your survivor's hand grasp is weakened, you may want to add lever handles or door lever adaptors to your door hardware.

Furniture and rugs. Now that you're inside, look around. Scatter rugs can pose a major problem to a stroke survivor who is unsteady on his feet. They should be removed, and any remaining carpets should be firmly secured to the floor. Keep in mind that carpet that's overly plush can be a drag on wheelchair mobility and a tripping hazard for someone using a walker.

Depending on your budget, you may want to buy furniture that moves up and down to accommodate a stroke survivor who has trouble standing up or sitting down. Mace says that there are furniture makers who incorporate these features into stylishly upholstered pieces that blend well with your home's decor. A bed that is too high or too low can be modified by either cutting down the legs or putting the whole thing on a platform. You might also want to rearrange furniture to make it easier for a stroke survivor to maneuver around the house, as well as to provide space in the living room so he doesn't have to sit outside the conversation area, suggests McGurran.

Kitchens. If your stroke survivor is in a wheelchair, you'll want to create as many open spaces as possible underneath spots like the sink and counters to allow the user to get closer to the cabinets. If that's not possible or such renovations are too expensive, a lot can be done by installing simple breadboards that slide in and out. They make great work surfaces, and you can even cut holes in them the size of your favorite bowl. Drop the bowl in the hole to help steady it.

Think creatively when it comes to the kitchen. Many wheelchair users can't operate a conventional stove because it's too high or the knobs are out of reach. McGurran suggests buying a small microwave for everyday use, rather than

Scatter rugs should be removed.

Will relocating faucets make them more accessible?

going to the expense of buying a new stove. And rather than buying a new sink, you can simply change faucet hardware to blade-type levers and/ or relocate faucets to the side of the sink instead of the back for easier use of the sink.

If you are committed to making renovations in the kitchen, consider buying a refrigerator with side-by-side refrigerator and freezer units, so that the person in a wheelchair has access to both the refrigerator and the freezer. And take advantage of pantry shelving, if you have it, to store food previously kept in high cabinets.

Bathrooms. Bathrooms can be a major source of problems, since so many of them are cramped, little spaces inaccessible to someone using a wheelchair or a walker. In addition, slippery surfaces can create a safety hazard. Before you undertake major remodeling, however, see if you can create more space by changing from a vanity to a wall-hung sink. Some people remove tubs and waterproof the floors to create roll-in showers and more maneuverability space for wheelchairs.

In addition to space considerations, you probably also want to add safety features such as grab bars for the toilet and tub areas, and a higher toilet seat if the survivor has trouble rising from a seated position. Bathroom fixtures like these are now available in attractive designs and materials, so you don't have to have a bathroom that looks like a hospital.

Grab bars for the toilet and tub areas are a must.

Special Products for Special People

When you're arranging to modify your home, you'll probably be introduced to the world of adaptive and assistive products for the disabled and physically challenged. An absolute wealth of ingenious products exists out there, but it can be an overwhelming job sorting through them.

For just about every task of daily living— from cooking and eating to bathing and groom-

There's a product made to help with almost every task of daily life.

ing—there's a host of products to aid a stroke survivor. You will be introduced to some of these products by occupational therapists while the survivor is still in the rehabilitation center. And therapists are invaluable in teaching survivors how to use such items to maximize their independence.

But after your survivor returns home and begins to adjust to daily life, you'll probably find yourselves needing and looking for other assistive items, not only to help in daily living activities but also to use when working, traveling, reading, writing and enjoying leisure time. These items can be tremendous morale boosters for your survivor, especially if they help him do something for himself that you used to have to help with. Or if they help him take part in an activity he thought he could no longer do, like playing cards with a card-holder designed for the person who has use of only one hand. There are many sources where you can find assistive items. Some devices—like nonskid tape for your stairs or bathtub—can be found in your local hardware or department store.

Hospital supply houses and direct mail catalogs offer invaluable aids.

Other, more specialized items—for those who have the use of only one arm or leg, or who have other stroke aftereffects like balancing problems—are usually available either through hospital supply houses or a growing number of mail-order catalogs that your rehab center or doctor can recommend. One person with a special interest in aids for daily living is Joan Ellen Foyder, the family caregivers' advocate who is the author of *Family Caregiver's Guide,* a book of practical, organizational advice. Foyder recommends that before you purchase anything, you check with your survivor's occupational therapist or other rehabilitation experts for advice on which aids are really the most helpful and suitable. "Try to arrange for the use of the actual article on trial before purchasing it," she advises. A picture could look perfect to your stroke survivor, but upon using it, he may find that it doesn't suit him.

Before you buy an assistive device, ask for a tryout.

One day when she was demonstrating a special pen for people with a limited ability to grasp, Foyder recalls, a woman in the audience thought the pen would be ideal. But upon trying it she realized immediately that it wouldn't help her particular problem. You could ask other stroke survivors in a support group if they've tried the item, or you could check it out at medical supply stores or home health care pharmacies, she says. If you do buy something by mail, be sure to ask about the company's return policy, especially if the aid is expensive.

But don't be afraid to pay a little more for an item your survivor will be using often, Foyder says. It can be cheaper in the long run because the item will last longer and look better. Why does it matter how it looks? Foyder says many stroke survivors and other disabled people may refuse to use self-help devices because they're afraid it will signal to the world that they're impaired.

Pay attention to how a device looks, or your stroke survivor may refuse to use it.

Some aids for daily living are really handsome and aesthetically pleasing in design, she says, and won't turn the survivor off because of an institutional look. A good example, is a button fastener, which can help a stroke survivor button and unbutton clothes. Lots of economical versions exist, she says, but there's a stylish Swedish model that looks like it belongs on a bedroom dresser.

Along with various catalogs, there are also several computerized retrieval systems which list assistive aids by category, like kitchen aids or dressing aids. People working on the system will help you locate a specific product. ABLEDATA is a service of the National Rehabilitation Information Center (NARIC), a government-funded resource center in Silver Spring, Maryland. It lists over 14,000 commercially available devices for rehabilitation and independent living. You pay $10 for up to 100 listings and $5 for each additional set of 100 listings.

Accent on Information, another system, also

Computer information systems can help, too.

lists products by category. It charges $12 for up to 50 items in a basic search and 8 cents for each additional listing. The charge for a search is waived, however, for any disabled individual who cannot afford to pay. Accent on Information is one of several services for disabled people produced by Cheever Publishing, Bloomington, Illinois. The company also publishes a magazine for the disabled, *Accent on Living*, which contains lots of product information.

Hiring Help: Home Care Resources

Home health care agencies can provide hands and wheels.

When Susan, a 58-year-old stroke survivor, came home from the rehabilitation hospital, her husband, Tom, hired Optional Care Systems, a private home health care agency based in St. Paul, Minnesota, to handle the services she would need. Because Tom worked, the agency arranged for a home health aide to come in 8 hours a day to care for Susan, prepare her meals and take care of the house. Three times a week, Susan received visits from a nurse, who checked her blood pressure.

In addition, physical and occupational therapists visited Susan three times a week to give her follow-up therapy. The home health aide helped Susan do the exercises and practice the skills that the therapists had recommended. Susan's insurance paid for all the services except the home health aide, which Tom and Susan had to pay for themselves.

At first you may need skilled health care workers.

You may be the principal caregiver at home, but especially in the beginning, your survivor may need the help of a variety of skilled health care and therapy providers if he is to continue making gains. And beyond those first days and months, depending on the situation, you may continue to need long-term homemaker services, especially if you work. Like Tom, you may choose a home health care agency to do all the work for you—screening, hiring, insuring, coordinating and finding out what funding sources may be available to you. But you can also coordinate services yourself, or use hospital-based or public health departments to help you obtain services.

The social worker or discharge planner at your rehabilitation hospital can often help you coordinate the home care you're going to need immediately after your stroke survivor returns home. He can put you in contact with community sources of care and help you sort through insurance policies to see what kind of home care is covered. As a general rule, most insurance policies will continue to pay for some medical and therapy services if your survivor's condition warrants.

A social worker can often help you coordinate the help you'll need.

But once he stops making what insurance companies term "progress" toward rehabilitation goals or reaches a level of "functional independence," many insurers cut off funding. A survivor who can walk with the help of a cane might be cut off from further physical therapy funding, for example, even though he could potentially progress to walking without a cane with further therapy.

Insurance payments may be cut off when the stroke survivor reaches "functional independence."

Insurers also stop paying for nursing services after a survivor reaches a level where they're no longer deemed necessary. And even when nursing and home health services *are* covered, it's only for a short time per day and often not every day. As in Susan's case, a nurse visited her only briefly three times a week. That leaves families to pay for what is called "custodial care"—the day-to-day homemaker and home health aide support that many stroke survivors still need. And, if you and your survivor believe he could still make progress and become even more independent, it's up to you to pay for physical, occupational or speech therapy after that point.

You should definitely get some help from a case management specialist in looking through the

A case manager from your county's social services department can guide you through the home care maze.

Nonprofit agencies may offer their services on a sliding scale basis.

maze of home care services and funding sources, the experts we talked to advise. Besides the help you can get from your rehabilitation center and from home health care agencies themselves, you can also hire a case manager through your county's social services department.

When you're hiring home care workers, there are several different kinds of agencies you can turn to. There are private home health care agencies, such as Optional Care Systems; hospital-based agencies; home care agencies offering mostly nonskilled homemaker help; nonprofit agencies, such as those connected with religious groups; and Visiting Nurse Associations, which can provide an array of home health services. The advantage of nonprofit agencies is that they often provide services on a sliding fee scale, so if your insurance doesn't cover a service you need, you may be able to negotiate a lower fee.

How do you know if the agency you've chosen is a good one? The National Association for Home Care recommends that you ask the agency the following questions.

- Is it certified by Medicare? This is one measure of quality, and one you must have if you're planning to pay for services through Medicare. However, this isn't the only measure of quality. If you're not using Medicare, you can rely on several other quality controls listed next.
- Is the agency licensed? Many states require licensing, usually through the state health department.
- Is the agency accredited? Several professional organizations accredit home health care agencies. The Joint Commission on Accreditation of Hospitals in Chicago accredits hospital-based agencies and free-standing home health agencies. The Na-

A good agency should be accredited by a professional organization.

tional League for Nursing in New York accredits nonprofit home health care agencies and skilled nursing services. The National Homecaring Council, a division of the Foundation for Hospice and Homecare in Washington, D.C., accredits homemaker/home health aide agencies.

- Does the agency provide written statements describing its services, eligibility requirements, fees and funding sources?
- How does the agency choose and train its employees? Does it protect them with written personnel policies, benefit packages and malpractice insurance?
- What's included in a nurse's or therapist's evaluation of your survivor's needs? Does he come to your home and consult with you and other family members? Does he consult with your survivor's doctor and other health professionals?
- Is the plan of care written out? Does it include specific duties to be performed, by whom, at what intervals and for how long? Can you review the plan?
- Does the plan allow you and other family members to be involved in understanding the care as much as possible?
- What are the financial arrangements? Can you get them in writing? Are there any extra charges?
- Does the agency send supervisors to visit your home and evaluate care regularly? Whom do you call with questions or complaints? Are your questions followed up and resolved?
- What arrangements are made for emergencies?
- What arrangements are made to ensure patient confidentiality?

Ask any home care agency if it provides a written plan of services.

- What plans and arrangements can be made for you if your reimbursement sources are exhausted?

Of course, you don't necessarily need to use a home care agency to find home care workers, especially if you're simply hiring someone to provide basic homemaker or home health aide services while you work or whenever you leave home. You can place a newspaper ad, get personal recommendations or use an employment agency, says Jean Crichton, author of *Age Care Sourcebook.*

Check references.

Be sure to check references, she advises, and take care that the homemaker/home health aide is a person with whom your survivor meshes well. You'll be an employer if you hire independently, and that means you have to pay wages and withhold taxes, supervise the worker, and have backup plans if the worker is sick, quits or is fired.

An efficient caregiver is a happy one.

For more information on home health care—how to find it, evaluate it and pay for it—there are several booklets available from the Foundation for Hospice and Homecare, 519 C Street NE, Stanton Park, Washington, DC 20002. You can also purchase through the foundation a copy of Joan Ellen Foyder's handy book *Family Caregiver's Guide.* Foyder not only tells you how to deal with home health care workers, she also provides a whole organizational plan, complete with charts and schedules (perforated for easy removal) for people who are providing care for a patient at home. Her belief, based on her own experience as a caregiver to her mother and as a professional consumer advocate, is that an efficient caregiver is a happier and less-stressed one.

Chapter 12

Your Stroke Survivor and You: Living One Day at a Time

You've had the ramp built, you've modified your home to make it easier for your stroke survivor to get around and do things, you've bought or rented the equipment you think you'll need and you've arranged for home health care to aid you in your caregiving tasks. The frantic, detail-filled days of planning are over and now your stroke survivor is home.

Having "graduated" from the formal rehabilitation program, your survivor is akin to the college or boot camp graduate who's been through basic training, but now needs experience in the field to get on with the business of living this renewed, post-stroke life. And it isn't easy, according to almost every one of the stroke survivors we interviewed.

Day-to-day improvements may be annoyingly small. Frustrations over what he still can't do or

It's a different life for everyone when a stroke survivor comes home.

**Day-to-day
improvements may be
small.**

say may be overwhelming. The aftereffects of a
stroke can be bafflingly complex, both for you and
for the survivor. Anger, the survivor's and your
own, may be a part of every one of these early
days, too. "Instead of being the father, the husband, the friend whom the family could lean on, I
was instead a totally immature adult-child, no
comparison to what I was before the stroke. I was
a new person that the family and friends didn't
want to see, but had to," writes Jim Meier, a stroke
survivor.

Different families have different "styles"—
ways they normally act and interact—that can be
particularly counterproductive when coping with
life after a stroke, says Hugh Carberry, Ph.D.,
chairman of the Psychology Department at Our
Lady of Lourdes Regional Rehabilitation Center in
Camden, New Jersey. If you recognize your family
style among these, modifying it might go a long
way toward easing tension at home.

The overprotective family. This family
never lets the survivor do anything for himself.

**Encourage the stroke
survivor to do things for
himself.**

Constantly doted on, the survivor quickly sees
himself as a "sick person" and becomes even more
dependent. But being that dependent makes the
survivor feel inadequate, and that inadequacy
makes him feel resentful of those who are always
doing everything for him. And the family quickly
becomes resentful, too, says Dr. Carberry, as they
rush around continuing to create the problem. The
lesson? Try as much as possible to let the stroke
survivor do for himself. Investigate self-help devices, such as those found in the catalogs we mentioned in chapter 11, to enhance that independence.

The underprotective family. This family is
still denying that the stroke survivor has disabil-

**But don't expect the
stroke survivor to do
everything he once did.**

ities, says Dr. Carberry. A typical example is when
the survivor is the mother of a family and the
family still expects her to do all that she did before.
But she just can't, and so she feels guilty and the
family feels resentful. This is especially trouble-

some if other family members have to take on new roles, like Dad having to cook. In this situation, families need to work together to realistically accept what the survivor can and cannot do. The survivor still needs to be pushed to try things, but within realistic limits, says Dr. Carberry.

The disorganized family. This family has very little structure and no defined roles. Family members eat, sleep, watch television and shop at unpredictable times, and no one takes definite responsibility for family activities. This can wreak havoc for the stroke survivor, who needs more structure in his life, especially if he has common stroke aftereffects like short- and long-term memory problems and a short attention span. Families need to build in regular meal times, sleep schedules and other routine daily activities to ease the anxiety the survivor may be feeling, says Dr. Carberry.

> A structured family life will help the stroke survivor.

The scapegoating family. This is an angry family, one whose members blame each other for all the things that go wrong, says Dr. Carberry. After a stroke occurs, the survivor can become the scapegoat—the family blames him for all that has gone wrong in their home. Or he, in turn, can blame everyone else for his difficulties.

One angry stroke survivor who wrote a letter to the editors of the *Stroke Connection* (a newsletter by and for stroke survivors published by the Courage Stroke Network—see the appendix, "The Family Caregivers' Resource Guide," for details) said his family was driving him to the point of another stroke because they argued and found fault with everything he did or said. Dr. Carberry says such families may need professional help to get over these intense feelings of hostility and reach a point where they can better adjust to what's happened to them.

> Families that blame their members for problems may need professional therapy.

Since anger can be part of a general state of depression, keep an eye out for other signs of depression in your survivor, like a loss of appetite, a lack of interest in therapy and a lot of crying and constant tiredness. Some of the survivors we inter-

> Keep an eye out for signs of depression.

viewed said that their depression hit not right after the stroke, but months later.

In chapter 9, we talked at length about post-stroke depression and how important it is to treat it with drugs, psychotherapy or a combination of the two. If a survivor's depression is allowed to go unchecked, it could really slow down his continuing rehabilitation gains. Experts in post-stroke depression say it could even trigger a kind of "pseudo-dementia," where the survivor feels like he is losing his mind. Don't hesitate to consult your doctor if you suspect your survivor is depressed.

Relearning Lost Skills

If your survivor has suffered a stroke that affects the left side of his body (meaning that the stroke occurred in the right side of his brain), there may be particularly irksome adjustment problems. These survivors are more likely to suffer from a short attention span, poor listening skills and short-term memory loss. So he may be harder to retrain in therapy sessions.

And these same problems, coupled with a loss of inhibitions (which leads survivors to say whatever they want, regardless of the effect on others) are even more troublesome in social situations. The survivor may offend others with too-forthright comments, a tendency to be self-centered or an inability to listen or follow conversations. If friends don't understand, you could lose important social supports, as people avoid visiting or conversing with your survivor.

Along with these problems, left-sided stroke survivors also tend to deny their deficits. You may find yourself arguing over using the car (which may be dangerous for a left-sided survivor, because of a loss of perceptual skills) and other unrealistic tasks they insist they can do. These same survivors may find it difficult to do everyday tasks, such as using a checkbook, dialing a telephone, putting

Stroke damage can sometimes cause people to say anything they want—without regard for its effect on others.

clothes on in the right order or following simple directions.

Dr. Carberry, who runs a highly respected retraining program for brain-injured adults, says there are many ways that families can help survivors recognize their deficits and compensate for them. "Many so-called memory problems we see in stroke survivors are really deficits in attention, concentration and organizational skills," he says. But the methods to help overcome these deficits involve memory-enhancing methods you may be familiar with.

You can overcome memory problems.

Survivors should practice repeating and reviewing things they want to remember, he says. If a survivor is introduced to a person, for example, he should "celebrate the name and spend some time talking about it. Ask about its ethnic origin or associate something familiar with the name," he says. Every survivor should keep a notebook, in which he plans the day ahead and records important information he'll need to use. If someone asks him a question and he can't remember the answer (such as a phone number or where he put the keys, for example), all the survivor needs to do is check the notebook.

Stroke survivors may find that repeating, recording and reviewing things will help them "remember."

Recording information in such a manner helps to retrain memory skills, says Dr. Carberry. "The stroke survivor should feel free to use the methods by which he learns best, whether it's writing things down, saying it out loud, forming a visual representation in the mind or a combination of these techniques."

You can also help your survivor learn to follow the sequence of tasks by writing directions down one step at a time—whether it's baking a cake or getting to a friend's house. Or you can review everyday tasks with the survivor and brainstorm about the steps he would use to solve particular problems. The tasks can be simple ones, such as how to choose and prepare a meal or how to buy furniture (first you find the names of furniture stores in the phone book, then you get in your

Write down directions one step at a time.

car and visit some shops, and so forth). By exercising the mind this way, the survivor is using and becoming familiar again with lost skills, says Dr. Carberry.

"I helped my kids with their baseball card collections," says Jerry Bigoness, a stroke survivor. "By sorting the cards, counting them and organizing them, I learned how to do those kinds of tasks again. And since I had trouble with reading, I used the cards for practice. There was so little to read on them, it made it easier for me."

Stroke survivors need to be encouraged to become more assertive about getting others to help them overcome their deficits, says Dr. Carberry. "Encourage them to ask questions or ask people to repeat things until they clearly understand what's being said," he advises. This assertiveness helps them become more involved with people again, too, he says.

> **Stroke survivors should demand that people repeat things until they understand what's being said.**

Because of the complexity of these kinds of stroke deficits, you may want to do some further reading about the effects of stroke. The American Heart Association (AHA) and the National Stroke Association (NSA) both publish excellent materials about stroke aftereffects, along with helpful suggestions on how survivors can practice to compensate for these problems.

In addition to single-sheet handouts and pamphlets, the NSA also publishes a book called *The Road Ahead: A Stroke Recovery Guide,* which is an impressively comprehensive resource for stroke survivors and their families. The book is filled with practical tips and strategies. In the appendix, we provide you with addresses for both associations.

As well as practicing to overcome cognitive and social deficits, your stroke survivor may also be attending physical, occupational and speech therapy sessions aimed at bringing him to a higher level of independence.

Physical therapists will probably continue to work with your survivor, encouraging him to improve strength, coordination and flexibility through a special exercise program that's been individually designed. Therapists will also work on specific goals with the survivor, such as improving walking skills, learning how to transfer to and from a bed or a toilet more efficiently and so on. Be sure you get a written copy of the survivor's exercise program and work with the therapist in learning the exercises. You and your fellow caregivers will be helping the survivor to exercise on days when therapy isn't scheduled and after formal therapy ends.

What if new problems surface or you think your survivor is making further gains and you want to upgrade his or her exercise program? Don't hesitate to get back in touch with your physical therapist, even if it's months after your insurance coverage for formal therapy ended, advises Peter Polga, director of physical and occupational therapy at the Courage Center. "Many survivors run into problems. They may develop more weakness in a limb, for example, or suffer lower backaches because of the way they are walking. We can work with them to develop new patterns of movement that can keep a problem from recurring. We can also teach them new stretching and strengthening exercises to try and solve the problem," he says.

Get back in touch with your therapist if new problems develop.

Sometimes, if your therapist feels that a program of formal therapy is warranted to work on new problems, your insurance company might pay for these additional sessions, says Polga. So don't shy away from contacting a therapist if you can't afford to pay for a long-term therapy program. Even if funding for an ongoing program is a problem, therapists can usually work with you to update your home program, he says.

If additional therapy is necessary, your insurance company may pick up the tab.

Along with physical therapy sessions, your survivor may also have occupational therapy sessions, especially as he settles in at home and discovers which activities of daily living need working on, says Jan Daly, supervisor of adult occupational therapy at the Courage Center. "Often, a survivor hears the principles of how to per-

Sometimes you don't know which daily activities need work until you get home and try them.

form daily tasks during formal rehabilitation, but when it comes to actually performing them at home, he may need extra help.

"Also, six months after a stroke, a survivor might be more ready to learn and practice kitchen or dressing skills," she says. "He or she may be psychologically more ready to hear it all." Daly says occupational therapists can perform home visits and advise you and your survivor on how to better set up the kitchen, for example, to accommodate the survivor's needs. "When survivors are learning how to perform tasks in their own homes, there's the natural advantage of being on your own turf," she says.

Along with practicing the tasks of daily living, an occupational therapist can also help your survivor perfect skills that will help him pursue hobbies, do volunteer work or return to a paying job, says Daly. "I'm working with a woman now on writing and typing, because those are the skills she needs to return to work."

An occupational therapist can help perfect skills.

Coping with Aphasia

Although exercising and practicing daily living skills like eating and dressing are important parts of a stroke survivor's days at home, probably nothing will concern you more than helping him regain speaking and language skills. If you're living with a survivor whose right side was affected by the stroke, chances are he is suffering from some degree of aphasia, the scrambling of the human communication system that can affect speech, comprehension of others' speech, reading, writing and gesturing.

Learning to communicate effectively again ranks at the top of most wish lists, according to aphasic survivors we interviewed. For without communication, the aphasic is trapped inside a mind that is still intelligent and functioning. It's just that the words won't come out, or others'

For an aphasic, the words won't come out— or they won't go in.

words are hard to process. "Intelligence and intellect are still there, it's just that the computer has gone down," says speech pathologist Norma Horwitch, founder and director of the Volunteer Stroke Rehabilitation Program in New Haven, Connecticut. This unique group of volunteers visits with aphasics to help them sharpen and practice language skills.

Whether a survivor has expressive aphasia, which means his main problems are in speaking and writing, or receptive aphasia, where the main problems are with understanding speech and reading, there is a lot you can do to keep his world stimulating. Making sure he's around people a lot and speaking frequently to him will frequently help an aphasic recover. It provides the kind of stimulation that may help him retrieve old language skills while learning new ones to overcome any problems he may still have. And when you've helped an aphasic communicate effectively again, you've offered him a "lifeline to sanity," in the words of aphasic Helen Wulf.

Just talking with a stroke survivor will help him recover his langauge skills.

If your survivor continues to get speech therapy after he returns home, make sure you continue to be a part of those sessions, too, advises Danbury, Connecticut, speech pathologist Carolyn B. Finch. You'll learn some of the methods speech pathologists use to help aphasics regain skills and you'll also learn how to reinforce those skills through practice programs at home.

There are also some basic dos and don'ts that you and other family members and friends of the aphasic should keep in mind, writes New York University speech pathologist Martha Taylor Sarno, M.D.hc, in her informative booklet, *Understanding Aphasia.* Here are a few.

Do: Encourage your aphasic to want to speak and take part in speech therapy. Praise even the most imperfect efforts and let him make mistakes while speaking. You can occasionally correct your aphasic, but too much criticism could make him retreat into silence, says Dr. Sarno. Give your

Keep communication short, simple and positive.

aphasic lots of opportunities to hear speech—television and radio can be good sources, too, if used sparingly. Keep your communication with him short and simple and speak slowly. Try repeating yourself if he doesn't understand. Keep a positive outlook and praise even the smallest gains your aphasic makes.

At the same time, be understanding of his frustration and tell him you sympathize with how difficult it must be. Treat your aphasic like an adult, even if he occasionally appears to be acting like a child. Along those lines, continue to include your aphasic in adult activities, like going to the movies, being with company and eating dinner with the family. This signals to your aphasic that you completely accept him as he is.

Do not talk for your aphasic.

Don't: Force your aphasic into therapy or into talking with people if he doesn't want to—forcing generally never works anyway. You shouldn't talk for him, either, when he is with other people, unless it's absolutely necessary. Along the same lines, don't interrupt him when he's trying to speak, even if his efforts are slow (which they often are). Talking for him or interrupting can quickly undermine his fragile self-confidence. Try not to scold or become irritated when your aphasic cannot communicate—it only makes things worse. Don't make big demands on him that he isn't prepared to meet.

Acknowledge the aphasic's difficulties in a tactful way.

You can help your aphasic's friends and family feel comfortable speaking with him again if you encourage them to follow a suggestion given to us by Catherine Caldarella Roberts, a Vermont nurse who has cared for patients with aphasia. "I always say 'I know it's difficult for you to speak—but go ahead.' Saying that always seems to break the ice between the aphasic and me." Acknowledging his difficulties in a tactful and sympathetic way may provide encouragement and reassure an aphasic that you're on his side.

Unfortunately, you and your aphasic survivor may find yourself all too soon facing the end of speech therapy services, as insurance funding runs out. If you're unable to afford more therapy sessions (most people aren't), it will be up to you to help your aphasic continue to improve his language skills. This is an enormous job and one for which the families of aphasics get very little community support. That's because the aphasic's needs are so specialized. Even stroke clubs, those reassuring groups of stroke survivors and their families who meet and support each other, don't often work out well for aphasics, because they have such trouble communicating—*especially* in a group.

Working with an aphasic is a demanding job.

But help is on the way, thanks to the efforts of dedicated people like Dr. Sarno, who is director of speech-language pathology at the Howard A. Rusk Institute of Rehabilitation Medicine, New York University School of Medicine. Dr. Sarno and fellow aphasia experts have started a National Aphasia Association (NAA) with several goals in mind. "We intend to stimulate the establishment of a network of clubs for aphasics and their families around the country," she says.

These clubs, which would be organized by speech pathologists and run locally, would give aphasics a chance to meet with each other in a supportive environment to practice their language skills. The NAA will support these groups with a manual about how to start an aphasia club. It will also provide the clubs and other interested individuals with educational materials and resources about aphasia.

The association's primary purpose is to educate the public about aphasia to counteract a popular belief that people who have lost their language skills are "crazy, or idiots, or dumb." Because aphasia is such a complex disorder, one in which recovery is often so difficult to understand or predict, Dr. Sarno says the association will also champion the unique needs of aphasics in the medical and rehabilitation communities, so that more and better services can be provided.

A new group will help people understand that aphasics are not "idiots."

The Volunteer Stroke Rehab Program sends volunteers to aphasics' homes.

In addition to the NAA, there's also the Volunteer Stroke Rehabilitation Program, which we mentioned earlier, where volunteers visit and spend time communicating with aphasics to help them regain language skills. The group, which has several chapters in Connecticut, would be happy to send its newsletter to those who request it. (For more information, see the box, "Community Stroke Aftercare Programs: Three Very Special Examples," on page 234.)

One newsletter provides a forum for aphasics.

There's also a wonderful newsletter by and for aphasics called *A Stroke of Luck.* It was started by Josephine Simonson, a speech pathologist, and Helen Wulf, an aphasic and author of a book about her struggles to regain language called *Aphasia, My World Alone.* Says Wulf: "*A Stroke of Luck* was designed to be a forum where aphasics and their families could vent frustration and share insights into their tricks of coping with aphasia and its strangeness. And, knowing they had a spot that was their own, we hoped it would lessen the dreadful loneliness many aphasics and their families feel."

Wulf says her readers, who have grown in number from 250 to 2,300 in less than five years, often write or call each other, which indicates to her that this kind of support system is needed. The newsletter is filled with incredible stories, as aphasics and family members tell of their struggles and victories, often with a touch of gentle humor. Sometimes an article will be written in the telegraphic, but definitely readable, prose of an aphasic who still cannot put complete sentences together. Letters almost always include the writer's name and address to aid readers' efforts to network with each other. This is an incredible resource, especially for people who may not have access to other aphasics or continuing speech therapy.

Another great contact for aphasics and their families who want to continue practicing language skills at home is speech pathologist Carolyn B. Finch, who has developed a low-cost correspondence speech therapy program, including audio/videotapes and testing materials. She will evaluate tapes of sessions you conduct with the aphasic and send you her comments.

Finch has also developed a unique emergency sign system called Universal Hand Talk: A Survival Sign System, which she has used successfully with aphasic stroke survivors who have not been able to learn to communicate through other means. The system can be learned in 4 hours, she says. (For more information on how to contact the National Aphasia Association, the Volunteer Stroke Rehabilitation Program, *A Stroke of Luck* and Carolyn Finch, see the appendix.)

You can even learn an emergency sign language through the mail.

Besides continuing to work on therapeutic recovery, survivors also need to reach out and make new social contacts. Along these lines, they may want to join stroke clubs and/or stroke support groups.

Think about encouraging your survivor to join a stroke club.

Stroke clubs are run by and for stroke survivors and their families. They give you new opportunities to make friends with people who've been down the road you're just starting on. Every stroke survivor we interviewed for this book spoke of the invaluable support stroke clubs gave them. Stroke survivors often lose old friends after their strokes, so the clubs become like a new social network for many.

Stroke clubs provide a new network of friends.

Stroke support groups, on the other hand, are usually run by rehabilitation professionals. They are more structured than clubs, as they focus more formally on helping you cope. But they, too, can be important sources of new friendship.

To locate a stroke club or support group in your area, start by asking members of your rehabilitation team. If you can't locate one, the NSA, the Courage Stroke Network or your local chapter of the AHA can often refer you to ones they've either sponsored or networked with. (All three groups' national addresses are listed in the appendix.)

Enjoying the Active Life

Although socializing is one form of recreation, you'll also want to encourage your survivor to get back into other recreational activities he used to enjoy. There are positively hundreds of self-help devices to entice survivors back to games and sports they loved, even if they have the use of only one hand or are in a wheelchair.

There's always a way to get back into sports and games.

"Survivors have to ask themselves what they want to do," says Lyn Rourke, supervisor of sports, physical education and recreation at the Courage Center. "Then you just problem-solve how to do it in a new way." The survivor's attitude is the biggest part of it, she says. "If he's enthusiastic, he can usually find a way to do just about whatever he wants."

How to encourage your survivor to want to get back into recreational activities? You've got to really "sell" your product with some sizzle, advises recreational therapist Dennis Dugan of Our Lady of Lourdes Regional Rehabilitation Center. "Make the activity really look like fun. Make it flashy." Dugan incorporates a lot of humor into the "selling" he does to his clients, and he emphasizes "having a good time."

Forget competition at first.

Along those lines, he encourages staying away from any heavy competition, especially at first. "Make sure to start by suggesting activities you know your survivor enjoyed before his stroke—they're usually a lot easier to do than new activities." And there's also the survivor's natural interest in familiar, enjoyable recreation. "One of the first things I wanted to do after I had my stroke was to knit," says stroke survivor Mary Balfour. "I've always loved knitting, and it was really important for me to do something I knew how to do before I had my stroke. I made lots of mistakes at first—but I did it!"

If your survivor's favorite activities involve two hands and he can use only one now, tell him about or demonstrate assistive devices that will help. If playing cards was his thing, for example, you can buy or make a card-holder so that he can still play. If fishing was his favorite outdoor sport, there are electric reels with batteries that retract the line while the survivor holds the rod with his strong hand, says Rourke.

Battery-powered reels make one-handed fishing a snap.

On the other hand, if your survivor's favorite form of recreation was something she really can't do anymore, try to encourage interest in new activities. Elaine Argetsinger, a stroke survivor who found she couldn't train her right hand to play the piano again, turned to art as a new form of creative expression. "I've had seven exhibits of art so far," she says proudly.

If your survivor was athletic before the stroke, or even if he was not, try to encourage participation in exercise activities. Staying active is a stress reducer for everyone, says Rourke, but it makes stroke survivors feel particularly good about themselves.

Exercise reduces stress.

The survivors we interviewed raved about swimming in particular, both as a relaxing activity and as one that helped them use the side of the body affected by the stroke. Many rehabilitation programs with access to a pool offer special classes where therapists help stroke survivors in the water. You might want to inquire if there are any such classes in your area.

Many stroke survivors rave about swimming.

There are also a number of exercise videotapes that have been produced for disabled people, such as *Nancy's Special Workout for the Physically Challenged*, produced by Nancy Sebring, an occupational therapist with a special interest in exercise. Sebring's workout is aerobic, that is, it gives your heart and lungs a workout—all from a seated position. She provides special instructions for stroke survivors and advises them how to adapt some of the two-handed exercises she demonstrates.

The Courage Stroke Network also offers an exercise tape expressly designed for stroke survivors. "We checked out the market on exercise tapes for the disabled and found that most of them included workouts that the average stroke survivor could not do," says coordinator Pat Kasell. "So we developed our own, which includes both flexibility and strengthening exercises." The tape features stroke survivors performing the exercises. (Information about how to obtain both tapes is in the appendix.)

Exercise videotapes show how to increase strength and flexibility.

If your stroke survivor was especially fond of outdoor sports, he might feel discouraged about whether he'll ever do them again. But he shouldn't, says John Kopchik, Jr., an outdoorsman who lost his leg in an auto accident. "He may be a little sloppier at casting and shooting—but he still can do it," Kopchik says.

One magazine is geared toward returning the outdoorsman to his natural habitat.

To encourage disabled sportsmen and provide them with a resource for information, Kopchik publishes and edits *Disabled Outdoors* magazine. In it, he motivates readers to try hunting, fishing, camping and boating again. There's information on accessible resorts and outfitters who acknowledge the needs of disabled hunters, plus details on new assistive products and special organizations, and how-to articles. This magazine could be just what your survivor needs to take up his sport again.

Survivors in wheelchairs who are interested in the booming world of wheelchair athletics might also enjoy *Sports 'N Spokes* magazine. Your survivor may never compete in the Boston Marathon (as some wheelchair athletes do), but he just might enjoy the upbeat spirit of the magazine while getting some ideas on how to keep exercising in a wheelchair.

Wheelchair sports are booming.

Another misconception that many stroke survivors and their families have is that they may never travel again because of the survivor's disabilities. But many train, plane and bus companies now offer special services for the disabled.

Whether you're planning an outdoor exercise activity or a week-long trip, it pays to check out your destination's accessibility, in terms of parking, buildings and restrooms, *before* you go, suggest the recreation experts we consulted. Nothing could ruin an activity more than not being able to get to it.

Check out your destination's accessibility before you go.

And finally, if your stroke survivor's disabilities keep him or her confined to home most of the time, don't despair. There are many games, hobbies and other recreational activities, which are therapeutic as well as challenging, to pass the time. The National Stroke Association recommends games like Mastermind, chess, checkers, Scrabble, Concentration and others for sharpening memory, perception, organization and problem-solving skills. If your survivor likes craft activities, these can also be therapeutic.

Board games can sharpen memory, perception, organization and problem-solving skills.

Don't forget art, music and photography, either. With special assistive equipment available from catalogs, these activities can liberate the mind. Other survivors continue to enjoy gardening, bird-watching and other nature pursuits. Birding could be particularly fun, especially if you live in a part of the country where many birds pass through as they migrate. Just keeping track of the birds, learning their names and classifying them can be a stimulating indoor hobby.

Along with these activities, encourage your survivor to write about his or her experiences. Pat Kasell, coordinator of the Courage Stroke Network, says writing seems to come naturally for stroke survivors she's met. And both the Stroke Network's *Stroke Connection* and Helen Wulf's newsletter *A Stroke of Luck* welcome and encour-

Encourage your stroke survivor to write about his experiences.

age written pieces from stroke survivors about their experiences.

Stroke survivor Mary Balfour got so interested in writing that she's been attending local classes to sharpen her writing skills. She has written 150 pages of a manuscript about stroke—both her experiences and medical aspects of the disease. Even if your survivor isn't interested in publishing, a journal or diary of events can be a rewarding, therapeutic, daily challenge.

If your survivor is interested and able to pursue volunteer or paid job opportunities, he should first identify interests, skills, talents, needs and goals, advises Mike Newman of the vocational services department at the Courage Center. "Does the survivor need a paycheck? Or does he or she need to be doing something productive?" Your survivor can contact a local vocational rehabilitation counselor about options for paid jobs, says Newman.

Your state should provide a local vocational rehab counselor to discuss job options.

Each state has a department or division of vocational rehabilitation staffed with counselors who coordinate and/or provide services which increase employment opportunities and promote greater independence for people with physical, cognitive or mental disabilities. In addition to the basic services of vocational counseling, planning, guidance and placement, special services may be available to clients, if needed. The rehabilitation center where your survivor stayed may also have vocational counseling.

Computers have revolutionized working at home.

But even if your survivor would have trouble finding transportation to a job or couldn't handle the demands of a full-time job, he might still be able to work at home or make other creative job arrangements. Many people with disabilities are finding work at home involving computers; and there's a special newsletter, *Computer Disability News*, published by the National Easter Seal Society in Chicago, that can keep you updated on advances in the use of computers by disabled people. Other stroke survivors team up and share a job.

One team of two included a man with poor speech skills, so he used the computer while his partner manned the phone.

If your survivor decides to pursue volunteer work, he should know that there's lots out there to be had, says Maureen Vanek of the Courage Center's volunteer department. You should contact your local United Way Volunteer Center for volunteering opportunities. Churches, schools and other nonprofit and volunteer groups are also usually in great need of volunteer help.

Volunteering can add structure to the stroke survivor's life, says stroke survivor and veteran volunteer Jeanette Weeks. "Working as a volunteer has provided me with structure, mental stimulation and challenges. I like the camaraderie of working with other people . . . My volunteer work has helped me regain my confidence and self-esteem," Weeks wrote in an article in the *Stroke Connection*."

A volunteer job can add structure to a stroke survivor's life.

One of the greatest ways to volunteer is to become a friendly visitor or peer counselor to other stroke survivors. (Check with your survivor's rehabilitation center to see if it can put you in touch with other survivors.) The Courage Stroke Network has a peer counseling program called Stroke Outreach, developed by stroke survivor Judy Hopia. Because she wished she'd had someone to talk to about her fears, frustrations and anxieties after her own stroke, Hopia thought other stroke survivors and their caregivers might benefit from such a program.

Become a visitor or counselor to other stroke survivors.

"If we could share our strengths and successes and tell all the newly stroke-involved about stroke groups, available literature on strokes and the adaptive aids that it took us so long to find, we feel it would be very encouraging," Hopia wrote in the *Stroke Connection* when she announced the formation of the program. She also felt that new stroke survivors would be encouraged seeing living

Stroke survivors can share their strength with new members of the "club."

(continued on page 280)

Paying for
Long-Term Home Care:
How Do Families Manage?

Thanks to Medicare and private insurance, most families don't have to worry much about paying for the hospital and rehabilitation center costs immediately surrounding a stroke. These "acute care" expenses are mostly covered. But later on, families face the cold, hard light of day when they find out how little of what are called "long-term care" expenses are paid by Medicare and most private insurance policies. Long-term care expenses can include everything from the homemaker you need to be with your survivor when you're not there through to the costs of modifying your home to make it accessible.

And those long-term care expenses can be considerable—even catastrophic in some cases. Even worse, they often come at a time when many families are experiencing a loss of income if the stroke survivor can no longer work. Even if they aren't catastrophic, such costs can still place an agonizing burden on a family's pocketbook.

Social workers and discharge planners at your rehabilitation center, counselors at your area office on aging and other case management specialists (who are found through nonprofit social service agencies, home health care agencies and other private agencies) can help you find and use other sources of funding for some of your other expenses. To pay for home modifications, for example, you may be able to obtain funds through community block development grants, deferred loan programs and/or other federal assistance programs, says Bruce Humphrys, head of the rehabilitation technology program at the Courage Center, Minneapolis.

But without the help of experts to find your way through the funding maze, you could be hopelessly overwhelmed. Many stroke survivors and their families ask themselves, "Why do we have to go through this tortuous process?"

Congressman Claude Pepper (D-Fla.), chairman of the House of Representatives Aging Committee's Subcommittee on Health and Long-Term Care, has been asking the same question for years. He and Congressman Edward R. Roybal (D-Cal.), chairman of the House Aging Committee, have written legislation that would provide Medicare coverage for comprehensive long-term care services provided in the home for disabled people like stroke survivors.

The legislation would provide for coverage of nursing care, homemaker/home health aide services, medical supplies and equipment, patient and family education and training, and case management services, among other things. The costs for this addition to the Medicare program would be entirely financed by lifting the income ceiling which dictates how much Americans are taxed for Medicare services. Under the new bill, they would be taxed up to the limits of their income. The bill's sponsors have shown how paying for long-term care at home can easily save millions of dollars compared with caring for people in nursing homes. For more information or to voice your support for the Medicare Long-Term Home Care Bill, contact the U.S. House of Representatives Select Committee on Aging, Subcommittee on Health and Long-Term Care, House Annex 2, Room 377, Washington, DC   20515.

proof that there is life after a stroke!

The Courage Stroke Network has now prepared a manual, describing how to start a peer counseling program, which it can send to any member of the network. If you and your survivor belong to a stroke club or want to start a peer counseling program in your area, you might want to write for this information.

Patience, humor and acceptance can make it all work.

A stroke survivor's days can be full ones, but to reach the point where that's possible most stroke survivors take millions of small steps along the way. Patience, a sense of humor and a gradually developed sense of acceptance of who they are now, stroke survivors tell us, are the ingredients that make it all work.

Appendix

The Family Caregivers' Resource Guide

Consider this your own personal guide to resources for life after a stroke. First there's a list of national stroke resource organizations, groups that provide a wealth of general information and support. Then there's a list of caregiver support sources—since you can't care for someone else until you care for you. There are also sources for help in modifying your home for a stroke-impaired person—especially for someone limited to the use of one side of his body.

And finally, there are lists of groups that help you cope, groups that help you understand, and groups that help you and your survivor regenerate your lives.

National Stroke Resource Organizations

American Heart Association
National Center
7320 Greenville Avenue
Dallas, TX 75231

The mission of the American Heart Association (AHA) is to eliminate all forms of cardiovascular disease and stroke. It publishes a variety of educational written materials about the prevention, treatment and rehabilitation of stroke. Its information about the risk factors for stroke is frequently the most up-to-date, since the AHA is intimately involved in research efforts. The pamphlets that explain the aftereffects of stroke can be particularly helpful if you're having trouble understanding all the complex changes you or a stroke survivor are going through. And some local AHA groups even sponsor stroke clubs for survivors and their families.

The AHA is also an excellent source of information on how to change your diet toward one that will help prevent strokes and heart disease. Depending on where you live, you could tap into their Culinary Hearts cooking programs (to teach you healthier cooking techniques), their dining-out programs (restaurants, airlines and hotels agree to serve menu selections which meet AHA guidelines for healthy meals) and other important community services.

Contact your local AHA unit (they're located all over the country) for information on how to find and use all these services.

Courage Stroke Network
Courage Center
3915 Golden Valley Road
Golden Valley, MN 55422

This is one of the most practical and useful national organizations for stroke survivors and their caregivers. Its focus is on the stroke survivor's life after he or she leaves the hospital or inpatient rehabilitation program. This is important, because it's often easier to make progress and keep your spirits up during a stay at a rehabilitation hospital.

That's where the Courage Stroke Network comes in. It offers crucial support to the stroke survivor after he or she gets on with living back at home. The network originated in Minnesota to provide a link between groups of stroke survivors who were meeting throughout Minnesota. It now networks with about 700 independent stroke groups throughout the United States, as well as with countless individual stroke survivors and their families. It is still based in Minneapolis and operated by the Courage Center, an organization providing innovative rehabilitation and independent living services to a variety of disabled people in the entire upper Midwest. These are among the network's many services.

Stroke group development. It promotes the formation of stroke groups—mutual help groups for people who have had stroke and their families. You can call their toll-free phone number from anywhere in the country to get information on an existing stroke group in your area. Or they'll help you start your own group. They'll even provide you with leadership training and educational materials to help get your group going.

Information and educational materials. A call to the network's toll-free number will also get you and your family educational materials on stroke, as well as referrals to other sources of information.

A newsletter by and for stroke survivors and their families. Tired of having people who haven't experienced a stroke or lived with a stroke survivor give you information? Then you'll love the *Stroke Connection*, the network's incredibly fine newsletter, written and edited mostly by stroke survivors and their families. In it, people share their personal experiences with stroke. They also offer tips, encouragement and help for continuing a productive life. This is useful as well as inspirational information. But it also seems to serve another purpose. It gives survivors and their families a forum for sharing their feelings about stroke—the frustrations, the anger, the positive changes and the growth. It's like a good group therapy session on paper. And you can contribute—the network welcomes letters and editorial contributions.

An exercise videotape for stroke survivors. The tape, *A Stroke Survivor Workout*, was developed after the network realized that most exercise tapes for the disabled weren't really practical for stroke survivors. This tape concentrates on strength and flexibility exercises, which can be therapeutically important for stroke survivors' muscles and joints.

Most of the services of the network are free or available at low cost.

National Stroke Association
300 East Hampden Avenue
Suite 240
Englewood, CO 80110

The National Stroke Association (NSA) was formed in 1984 as a national advocate for stroke survivors and their families. The NSA provides a variety of well-written educational materials on stroke prevention, medical treatment, rehabilitation, socialization and long-term care. Along with pamphlets and fact sheets, NSA publishes an excellent book for stroke survivors and caregivers, called *The Road Ahead: A Stroke Recovery Guide.* The book contains a wealth of information on living with the aftereffects of stroke. There are great tips for how to set goals for continuing therapeutic, recreational and social activities, plus lots of good, easy-to-read basic information on all aspects of stroke.

The NSA also publishes a quarterly newsletter, *Open Channels,* and runs a national clearinghouse which survivors and their families can call or write to get more information and referrals. The clearinghouse can, for example, refer you to a stroke club or support group in your area, or refer you to a local rehabilitation center. "We can answer all kinds of questions," says Karin Schumacher, director of program development. The NSA is also working to develop local chapters and raise money for research. For information on how to order written materials, contact the association at its address above.

Caregiver Support

Children of Aging Parents
2761 Trenton Road
Levittown, PA 19056

Children of Aging Parents (CAPS) provides a variety of supportive services for caregivers. When you join, you get two newsletters, *The CAPSule* and *Advice for Adults with Aging Parents or Dependent Spouses.* You also can contact them to find a caregivers support group in your area. If there's none around, CAPS will help you start one, with a start-up packet of materials. The group also provides general information and referral services to help you network with other caregivers.

National Council on the Aging Family Caregivers
   of the Aging Program
600 Maryland Avenue SW, West Wing 100
Washington, DC 20024

The National Council on the Aging (NCOA) started its membership group program for family caregivers because it was getting so many calls for help from caregivers all over the country. When caregivers join, with their membership fee comes a newsletter called *Caregiving,* plus other information on a variety of topics of interest to caregivers, especially on taking care of themselves. The program also sells guidebooks for starting a caregiver support group and information on legal and financial planning, respite care and other topics. It also sells two series of pamphlets for caregivers. One series is called *Family Homecaring Guides,* and the other is the *Caregiving Tips* series. You can also call the program to get a referral to a caregivers' support group in your area.

Adapting Your Home

Barrier Free Environments, Inc.
P.O. Box 30634
Water Garden, Highway 70 West
Raleigh, NC 27622

This architecture and design firm specializes in design for disabled and older people. It offers books and guides on how to adapt various parts of your home for a disabled person, including specifications and drawings which your local builder could follow.

Why would he need this kind of guidance? Most local builders don't know the best and safest ways to modify homes for the disabled, according to several experts we consulted. If you were planning to make major changes in your home, Barrier Free Environments could act as a consultant, with plans that a local builder could carry out. The firm also could refer you to a specialist in barrier-free design in your area or simply answer any questions you may have.

Paralyzed Veterans of America
801 Eighteenth Street NW
Washington, DC 20006

Paralyzed Veterans of America offers illustrated guides—including specifications—which you can pass on to builders who are helping you modify your home for a stroke survivor. It also offers individual tips and hints that you can use in making small, simple adaptations to your home.

Stroke Survival

Recreational Resources

Disabled Outdoors
John Kopchik, Jr., editor and publisher
5223 South Lorel Avenue
Chicago, IL 60638

This is a quarterly magazine for a stroke survivor who's interested in hunting, fishing, camping and boating, despite a disability. "You can do it!" says editor and publisher John Kopchik, who was himself disabled after an auto accident. The magazine is filled with tips and hints on how you can get back to the outdoors, products for making it easier and recreational locations that are accessible to those with disabilities.

Don Krebs' Access to Recreation
2509 East Thousand Oaks Boulevard, Suite 430
Thousand Oaks, CA 91362

This is a catalog filled with adaptive recreation equipment for people who are physically challenged. It contains everything from weight machines and specially equipped wheelchairs to swimming aids, camera equipment and fishing paraphernalia.

Nancy's Special Workout for the Physically Challenged
P.O. Box 2914
Southfield, MI 48037-2914

This exercise videotape is truly aerobic, and all the exercises are performed from a seated position. Occupational therapist Nancy Sebring is the instructor and she's a real motivator. Sebring also includes some special instructions for stroke survivors, who may not be able to perform some of her two-handed exercises. (The Courage Stroke Network also produces an exercise videotape designed for stroke survivors. See the network's listing in the section on National Stroke Resource Organizations.)

Stroke Clubs

Information on how to find or start a stroke club in your area can be obtained from the Courage Stroke Network, the National Stroke Association and local chapters of the American Heart Association. (See National Stroke Resource Organizations section for addresses.) These self-supporting groups give immeasurable support to stroke survivors and their families and provide a real link back to social activities.

Supportive Services for Aphasics

A Stroke of Luck
Helen Wulf
9305 Waterview Road
Dallas, TX 75218

A Stroke of Luck is an inspiring newsletter by and for aphasics and their families, edited by aphasic Helen Wulf. This is a real written lifeline for survivors and those who live with them. Readers who write in the newsletter often include their addresses. Then other readers can get in touch with them through the mail or over the phone.

Carolyn B. Finch
Bogart Communications
51 Cedar Drive
Danbury, CT 06811

Finch, who is a speech/language pathologist, has a low-cost correspondence and tape program for speech/language therapy so that families can continue to help aphasics try to make gains even after the period of professional therapy ends. You can record an audiotape or audiovisual tape of your speech and language work with the survivor, mail it to her at the above address and she'll evaluate it for you. Finch has also devised a sign system called Universal Hand Talk: A Survival Sign System, for people to use when other forms of communication aren't possible. She has used the system successfully with aphasics who haven't been able to communicate any other way. The system of 48 hand signs is easy to learn and is available on both audio- and videotapes. Posters, wallet cards and a pocket-sized guidebook reinforce the system.

National Aphasia Association
400 East Thirty-fourth Street, Room RR306
New York, NY 10016

This is an organization devoted to publicizing the needs of aphasics as well as to providing education, written information and support to the families of aphasics. The association supports the formation of special clubs for aphasics across the country, where they can go in a nonthreatening atmosphere and spend time socializing and practicing their language skills. Clubs network with each other through the National Aphasia Association. The association also educates a public unfamiliar with aphasia with information about the language disorder, so that aphasics will be treated with more understanding.

Volunteer Stroke Rehabilitation Program, Inc.
96 Westwood Road
New Haven, CT 06515

The Volunteer Stroke Rehabilitation Program (VSRP) is a regional program, but it invites inquiries about starting other chapters from families of aphasics and others interested in helping aphasics. VSRP volunteers visit aphasic stroke survivors in their homes and spend time talking with them and doing other activities. Each survivor is visited by two or three volunteers a week. The volunteers provide stimulating conversation and activity—giving aphasics the opportunity to practice their language skills and hopefully regain some of their lost proficiency. In the process, aphasics are relieved of some of the boredom and isolation they feel because they've lost the ability to communicate efficiently with others. The program—which is free—is effective as a complement to formal speech/language therapy, and it's a way to keep practicing language skills after formal therapy comes to an end.

INDEX

Anticoagulant medication. *See
   also specific medications*
   irregular heartbeat and, 167
   stroke prevention and,
      157–59, 167
Antidepressant drugs, 214
Aphasia, 11–12, 206–11
   categories of, 12
   coping with, 266–72
   correspondence speech ther-
      apy program for, 271
   emergency sign system for,
      271
   expressive, 209
   global, 209
   help organizations, 269–70
   receptive, 209
   supportive services for,
      287–89
ARISE, 234–36
Arteriogram, 173
   in mini-strokes, 52–53
Artery(ies)
   clogged, 171
   damaged, 19–20
   high blood pressure and,
      19–20
   noisy, 30–31
Artificial sweeteners, 87
Aspirin
   availability of, 160
   benefits of, 160
   blood clots and, 152–53
   dosage of, 155–56
   heart attack and, 153
   interactions of, 160
   negative effect of, 154
   noisy arteries and, 156–57
   platelet sensitivity to, 154
   positive effect of, 154
   precautions for, 160–61

risk of stroke and, 153–54
side effects of, 160–61
after TIA, 153–54
uses of, 160
Assertiveness, 264
   in caregiver, 232
Atherosclerosis, 6
   diet and, 58–59
Atrial fibrillation, 23–24
Aversive smoking, as smoking cessation technique, 140

B
Barrier Free Environments, Inc.,
   248–49, 285–86
Beans
   cooking with, 91
   fat calories in, 77
Bedsores, 198
Beef, fat calories in, 75
Bicycling, 121–23
   beginner's program, 122
   stationary, 121
Blindness, as indication of TIA,
   47–48
Blocked arteries, 172–74
Blood cholesterol levels, 36–40
   exercise and, 103–4
   high, 24–25
Blood clots, exercise and, 104
Blood pressure, 19. *See also* Hypertension
   diastolic, 36
   exercise and, 103
   home measurement of, 20–21
   physical inactivity and, 103
   readings of, 36
   salt and, 60
   systolic, 36
Blood sugar tests, 41–42
Blood test, 36

Grain(s)
    fat calories in, 77
    fiber in, 92
Grieving, 212

H
Handicapped. *See* Stroke survivor(s)
HDL. *See* High-density lipoprotein (HDL) cholesterol
Health
    blueprint for, 33–36
    recipes for, 96
Heart. *See also specific heart diseases*
    cookbooks for prevention of diseases of, 97
    enlarged, 19
    high blood pressure and, 19
    risk of stroke and, 22–24
Heartbeat. *See* Heart rate
Heart rate. *See also* Target heart rate
    during exercise, 106–7
    irregular, 23–24
        anticoagulant medication and, 167
Hemorrhagic stroke, 7
Heparin
    availability of, 164
    brand names of, 164
    interactions of, 164–65
    precautions for, 165–66
    side effects of, 164–66
    uses of, 164
Herbs, 84–85
High blood pressure. *See* Hypertension
High-density lipo-protein (HDL) cholesterol, 39-41
High-fiber foods, 63–64

Home blood pressure machine, 20–21
Home health care
    agencies, 254–58
        recommendations for, 256–58
    long-term, paying for, 278–79
Home modifications, 247–58
    bathrooms, 251
    entrances, 249–50
    exits, 249–50
    furniture, 250
    information on, 248–49
    kitchens, 250–51
    ramp, 248
    resources for, 285–86
    rugs, 250
    special products, 251–54
        assistive devices, 252–53
        button fasteners, 253
        computer information systems and, 253–54
    temporary, 247–48
    shower, 248
Humiliation, 208
Hypertension, 18–22. *See also* Blood pressure
    arteries and, 19–20
    control of, 21–22
    detection of, 36
    effects of, 19
    exercise and, 103
    heart and, 19
    physical inactivity and, 103
    salt and, 60
    stepped care in, 22
    undetected, 20–21
Hypertrophy, 23
Hypnosis, as smoking cessation technique, 139–40

Vision, distorted, as indication of
TIA, 47–48
Volunteer Stroke Rehabilitation
Program (VSRP), 238–40,
288–89

W
Walking, 109–14
blood pressure and, 110
calories burned by, 110–11
cardiovascular disease and,
109
gradual approach to,
112–13
indoor, 128
making time for, 113–14
program for, 117–18
shoes for, 111–12
technique to, 113
treadmills, 123–24
weight loss and, 110–11
Warfarin. *See* Coumarin

Weakness, as indication of TIA,
46
Weight chart, 62
Weight-loss, 92–100
assertiveness and, 98
discouragement and, 98–99
eating habits and, 95
control of, 94–95
enjoyment of, 99–100
exercise and, 104–5
failure and, 100
food diary for, 94
meal-planning and, 98
plateaus in, 98–99
walking and, 110–11
Weight training, 105. *See also* Exercise
Wolf, Philip A., 16, 17, 18,
25–26, 29–30, 32

Y
Yogurt, 81–82